Imaging for Students

David A Lisle, FRACR

Consultant Radiologist, Holy Spirit
Hospital, Brisbane, Visiting Radiologist,
Royal Brisbane and Children's Hospitals,
Lecturer in Anatomy and Radiology at the
Queensland University of Technology and
Clinical Lecturer in Radiology at the
University of Queensland Medical School,
Brisbane, Australia

With contributions by
Ken Mitchell, FRACR

Consultant Radiologist, Princess Alexandra
Hospital, Brisbane
Visiting Radiologist, Royal Brisbane
Hospital, Brisbane, Australia

and
Andrew Russell, FANZCA

Consultant Anaesthetist,
Holy Spirit and Princess Alexandra
Hospitals, Brisbane, Australia

ARNOLD

A member of the Hodder Headline Group
LONDON • SYDNEY • AUCKLAND
Co-published in the USA by
Oxford University Press, Inc., New York

First published in Great Britain 1996 by
Arnold, a member of the Hodder Headline Group
338 Euston Road, London NW1 3BH

Second impression 1997

Co-published in the United States of America by
Oxford University Press, Inc.,
198 Madison Avenue, New York, NY 10016
Oxford is a registered trademark of Oxford University Press

Whilst the advice and information in this book is believed to be true and
accurate at the date of going to press, neither the author nor the publisher
can accept any legal responsibility or liability for any errors or omissions
that may be made. In particular (but without limiting the generality of the
preceding disclaimer) every effort has been made to check drug dosages;
however, it is still possible that errors have been missed. Furthermore,
dosage schedules are constantly being revised and new side effects
recognized. For these reasons the reader is strongly urged to consult the
drug companies' printed instructions before administering any of the drugs
recommended in this book.

British Library Cataloguing in Publication Data
A catalogue record for this book is available from the British Library

Library of Congress Cataloging-in-Publication Data
A catalog record for this book is available from the Library of Congress

ISBN 0 340 61383 1

Typeset in 10/12pt Plantin by Scribe Design, Gillingham, Kent
Printed and bound in Great Britain by The Bath Press, Bath

Imaging for Students

Contents

Preface   vi
Acknowledgements   vii

Section I Introductory topics
1. Conventional Radiography – X-rays; plain films   *1*
2. Radiological hazards and protection   *4*
3. Intravascular contrast media   *7*
   Andrew Russel

Section II Plain-film interpretation
4. Chest X-ray   *10*
5. Abdomen X-ray   *41*
6. Skull X-ray   *51*

Section III Imaging techniques
7. Radiological procedures   *58*
8. Interventional radiology   *71*
   Ken Mitchell
9. Ultrasound   *78*
10. Computed tomography (CT)   *81*
11. Scintigraphy – nuclear medicine   *85*
12. Magnetic resonance imaging (MRI)   *89*

Section IV Imaging in clinical practice
13. Cardiovascular system   *95*
14. Respiratory system   *104*
15. Gastrointestinal tract   *109*
16. Urinary tract   *118*
17. Female reproductive system   *126*
18. Skeletal system   *131*
19. Central nervous system   *142*
20. Investigation of spine disorders   *149*
21. Paediatrics   *158*
22. Staging of malignancy   *166*
23. Imaging of AIDS   *171*

Index   177

Preface

Eine Neue Art von Strahlen (On a New Kind of Rays) was the title of the first publication on X-rays, written by Wilhelm Conrad Roentgen, and it appeared in the 1895 Annals of the Würzburg Physical Medical Society. A few weeks earlier, in November 1895, Roentgen had discovered X-rays. As such, 1995 marks the centenary of the birth of the speciality of Radiology. Since 1895, and particularly since 1960, there has been a proliferation of imaging technologies including ultrasound, CT, scintigraphy (nuclear medicine), and MRI. Unfortunately, teaching in Radiology in most medical schools has failed to keep pace with these developments. This publication fulfils the need for a book on imaging directed specifically at medical students.

The book has been set out in four sections and 23 chapters in what, I hope, gives a logical introduction to the subject of medical imaging.

Section I deals with introductory topics. A brief explanation of X-rays is followed by chapters on radiation hazards and protection and intravascular contrast media. The importance of recognising and treating contrast media reactions cannot be understated. Dr Andrew Russell, a consultant Anaesthetist, addresses these topics in some detail.

Section II deals with plain film interpretation. The chapter on chest X-rays is the longest in the book, underlining the importance of this topic. Abdomen and skull X-rays are also covered in this section. Spine and other skeletal X-rays are addressed in Section IV.

Section III covers imaging techniques including the newer modalities of ultrasound, scintigraphy, CT, and MRI. A chapter on radiological procedures is included to give medical students an overview of what is involved with each of the more common procedures including patient preparation, post-procedure observations and care, and complications which may occur. This section includes the chapter on interventional radiology prepared by a specialist in this field, Dr Ken Mitchell.

The use of imaging in clinical practice is discussed in Section IV. Under each system imaging investigation of the more common clinical problem is discussed. In an effort not to duplicate material covered elsewhere, the chapter on skeletal radiology covers only selected topics.

A chapter on AIDS is included due to the unfortunate increase in the incidence of this terrible disease. In reading these chapters medical students must keep in mind that imaging practices will vary according to geographical and economic circumstances. Whilst MRI and other high-technology techniques are readily available in Western society, a large percentage of the world's population has no access to these modalities.

Acknowledgements

Many people have given me invaluable assistance with this project. I would like to thank the following friends and colleagues who donated images, proof-read chapters, and generally gave help and support:

Dr Pat Carroll
Dr John Earwaker
Dr Julian Egerton-Vernon
Dr Frank Gardiner
Dr Sutherland MacKechnie
Dr Anthony Murphy
Dr John Ratcliffe
Dr Jane Reasbeck
Dr Richard Slaughter

In particular, I must thank Drs Ken Mitchell and Andrew Russell for their contributions to this book. They cheerfully and promptly interrupted their busy schedules in response to my requests for help and this is greatly appreciated.

Finally, my thanks go to Mrs Beverley Cook, Miss Esther Dragt, and Mrs Karen McHugh for typing and setting out the manuscript. As a computer illiterate, I owe them a huge debt of gratitude.

DEDICATION

To my parents
Ron and Shirley

and my sisters
Trina and Sallyanne

SECTION I
Introductory topics

1

Conventional radiography – X-rays; plain films

A. Conventional tomography

X-rays are a form of electromagnetic radiation; their frequency and energy are much greater than visible light. X-rays are produced in an X-ray tube by focusing a beam of high-energy electrons on to a tungsten target. They are able to pass through a patient and on to X-ray film thus producing an image (Fig. 1.1).

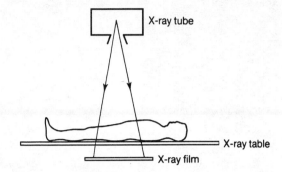

Fig. 1.1   Conventional radiography.

In passing through a patient the X-ray beam is decreased according to the density and atomic number of the various tissues through which it passes in a process known as *attenuation*. X-rays turn X-ray film black. Therefore the less dense a material, the more X-rays get through and the blacker the film, i.e. materials of low density appear darker than objects of high density.

Five principle densities are recognised on plain X-ray films. They are listed here in order of increasing density:

1. Air/gas: *black* (e.g. lung, bowel, stomach).
2. Fat: *dark grey* (e.g. subcutaneous tissue layer, retroperitoneal fat).
3. Soft tissues/water: *light grey* (e.g. solid organs, heart, blood vessels, muscle, fluid-filled organs such as bladder).
4. Bone: *off-white*.
5. Contrast material/metal: *bright white* (Fig. 1.2).

An object will be seen with conventional radiography if its borders lie beside tissue of different density. For example, the right heart border is seen because it lies against aerated lung which is less dense; should that part of the lung (right middle lobe) be collapsed or consolidated, it then has soft tissue density and the right heart border is no longer seen. Similarly, the psoas muscle

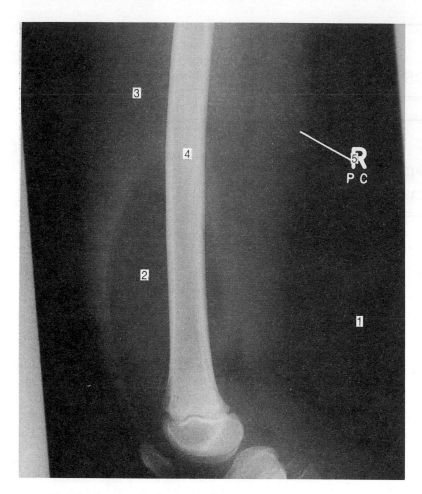

Fig. 1.2   The five principal
radiographic densities. This plain
film of a benign lipoma in a child's
thigh demonstrates nicely the 5
basic radiographic densities:
1. air
2. fat
3. soft tissue
4. bone
5. metal

margin is seen on a plain abdominal film owing
to the lower density of fat lying against it;
retroperitoneal fluid or soft tissue mass lead to
loss of visualisation of the psoas margin. These
comments apply to all radiographically visible
anatomical interfaces in the body.

A. CONVENTIONAL TOMOGRAPHY

Conventional tomography or *sectional radiography*
may be used where an object is obscured by
overlying or underlying structures. A good
example is during IVP where the kidneys may be
obscured by overlying bowel loops.

With conventional tomography, the X-ray tube
and X-ray film move about a pivot set at a
desired level of interest. Objects above and below
the plane of pivot are blurred by the motion of

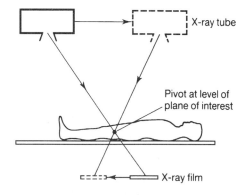

Fig. 1.3   Conventional tomography.
The X-ray tube and X-ray film move about a pivot, the
level of which is set at the desired plane of interest.

tube and film, while objects in the plane of interest are seen in sharper relief (Fig. 1.3).

Conventional tomography is used less in
modern practice since the advent of cross-

sectional imaging techniques (ultrasound, CT, MRI), though it still finds application in IVP, as above, and in some complex orthopaedic problems.

Further Reading

1. Curry TS, Dowdy JE, Murray RC (eds). *Christensen's Physics of Diagnostic Radiology*, 4th edn. Lea and Febiger, 1990.

2. Keats TE. *Atlas of Normal Roentgen Variants that May Simulate Disease*, 5th edn. Mosby Year Book, 1992.

3. Sutton D. (ed.). *A Textbook of Radiology and Imaging*, 4th edn. Churchill Livingstone, 1987.

4. Weir J, Abrahams PH (eds). *An Imaging Atlas of Human Anatomy*, 3rd edn. Wolfe Publishing, 1992.

2

Radiological hazards and protection

A. Radiation hazards
B. Protection in radiological practice

The International Commission on Radiological Protection (ICRP) was set up in 1928. It consists of expert delegates from many countries and its recommendations are accepted as worldwide standards. This chapter is a summary of numerous ICRP publications and recommendations on radiation hazards and protection, as well as recommendations of the National Health and Medical Research Council of Australia.

A. RADIATION HAZARDS

Radiation hazards occur as a result of damage to cells caused by radiation. This damage takes many forms:

- Cell death.
- Mitotic inhibition (temporary/permanent).
- Chromosome damage/genetic damage leading to mutations.
- Actively dividing cells are particularly sensitive (i.e. bone marrow, lymph glands, gonads).

The nature and degree of cell damage vary according to:

- Radiation dose.
- Dose rate.
- Irradiated volume.
- Type of radiation.

In general, two types of effects are seen as a result of radiation damage:

1. Stochastic effects

- Probability of effect, not severity, regarded as a function of dose.
- No dose threshold below which an effect will not theoretically occur.
- Due to modified cell, e.g. somatic cell leading to cancers; reproduction cell leading to hereditary effect.

2. Deterministic effects

- Severity of effects varies with dose.
- Dose threshold may exist below which the effect will not occur.
- Due to cell death, deterministic effects occur when cell loss is sufficient to impair organ function (e.g. radiation burns, cataracts, decreased fertility).

Units of radiation dose:

I. Absorbed dose

- Absorbed dose refers to the amount of energy imparted by ionising radiation in a given mass of matter.
- The SI unit is Joules per kilogram (i.e. J kg^{-1}) and is referred to as the Gray (Gy): 1 Gy = 1.0 J kg^{-1}.

2. Dose equivalent

- The concept of dose equivalent takes into account the fact that some kinds of radiation can produce more damage in tissue than others, even though the absorbed dose may be the same.
- Weighting factors are used for various radiation types, as below:

Photons, i.e. X-rays Gamma rays	1
Electrons	1
Neutrons	5–20
	depending on energy
Protons	5
Alpha particles	20

- Equivalent dose = weighting factor × absorbed dose
- The SI unit is Joules per kilogram, (i.e. J kg^{-1}) and is referred to as the Sievert (Sv): 1 Sv = 1.0 J kg^{-1}.

Examples of typical doses to an adult patient for some common X-ray procedures are:

Dose per film (mGy = 0.001 Gy)

	Skin	Bone marrow	Ovary
Abdomen AP	4.9	0.48	0.84
Chest PA	0.2	0.042	0.002
Pelvis AP	4.0	0.530	0.75
IVP	5.2	0.47	0.53
Lumbar lateral Spine	20.7	0.79	1.36

Examples of typical doses to an adult patient from some common nuclear medicine studies are:

	Total body dose equivalent (mSv)
Thyroid scan ^{99m}Tc	11.6
Bone scan ^{99m}Tc-MDP	5.2
Lung scan ^{99m}Tc-MAA	1.8
Gallium scan ^{67}Ga	20.3

Total average intake from natural background radioactivity, including cosmic and terrestrial radiation, is 1–2 mSv per year.

In considering the concept of detriment caused by radiation exposure, four factors are considered:

1. Probability of developing a fatal cancer.
2. Probability of developing a non-fatal cancer.
3. Probability of severe hereditary effects.
4. Length of life lost if harm occurs.

Based heavily on studies of Japanese survivors of atomic bomb attacks, ICRP-calculated probability coefficients for stochastic effects in the general population are as follows:

Detriment (10^{-2} Sv^{-1})	
Fatal cancer:	5.0
Non-fatal cancer:	1.0
Severe hereditary effects:	1.3
Total	7.3

e.g. if 100 people are exposed to 1 Sv of radiation, 5 will theoretically develop a fatal cancer. A dose of 5–6 Sv over a short time period leads to acute radiation sickness and death.

B. PROTECTION IN RADIOLOGICAL PRACTICE

Aims and principles of radiation protection are:

1. To prevent deterministic effects.
2. To limit the probability of stochastic effects by keeping all justifiable exposure *as low as is reasonably achievable* (ALARA principle): this includes keeping as low as possible doses to individuals, the number of people exposed, and the liklihood of others being exposed.
3. No practice is adopted unless its introduction produces a benefit which outweighs its detriment, i.e. positive net benefit.

With these aims and principles in mind, the following guidelines are used for radiographic procedures.

1. Protection of patient

- Each exposure justified on a case-by-case basis.
- Minimise number of X-ray films taken.
- Minimise screening time.
- Focus beam accurately to area of interest.
- Only trained personnel to operate equipment.
- Good equipment to be used, including rare earth screens, adequate filtration of X-ray beams, etc.
- Minimise the use of mobile equipment.
- Use ultrasound or MRI where possible.
- Quality assurance programmes in each department, including correct installation, calibration, and regular testing of equipment.

2. Paedatrics

- Special attention to minimising number of exposures, screening times, and the use of well-focused beams.
- Use of restraining devices and/or sedation.
- Gonad shields.
- If parents are required in the room, they should wear lead coats and not be directly exposed to radiation.

3. Women of reproductive age

- Minimise radiation exposure of abdomen and pelvis.
- Consider any woman of reproductive age whose period is overdue to be pregnant.
- Ask all females of reproductive age if they could be pregnant.
- Post-multilingual signs in prominent places asking patients to notify the radiographer of possible pregnancy.

4. Pregnancy

- As organogenesis is unlikely to be occurring in an embryo in the first 4 weeks following the last menstrual period, this is not considered a critical period for radiation exposure.
- Organogenesis commences soon after the time of the first missed period and continues for the next 3–4 months; hence during this time the foetus is considered to be radio-sensitive.
- Examination of the abdomen or pelvis should be delayed if possible to a time when foetal sensitivity is reduced, i.e. post-24 weeks' gestation (or ideally until the baby is born).
- Where possible, ultrasound or MRI should be used.
- Exposure to remote areas (e.g. chest, skull, limbs) may be undertaken with minimal foetal exposure at any time during pregnancy.
- Lead aprons draped over the abdomen are more reassuring than of practical value.
- Nuclear medicine studies are best avoided if possible during pregnancy.
- For nuclear medicine studies in the post-partum period, it is advised that breast-feeding be ceased and breast milk discarded for 2 days following the injection of radionuclide.

5. Protection of staff (including medical students!)

- Only necessary staff to be present in a room where X-ray procedures are being performed: TV monitors placed outside the screening room usually mean that students may observe procedures at a safe distance.
- Staff to wear protective clothing (e.g. lead aprons).
- At no time should staff be directly irradiated by the primary beam: lead gloves must be worn if the hands may be irradiated (e.g. in immobilising patients or performing stress views).
- All X-ray rooms should have lead lining in their walls, ceilings, and floors.

Further Reading

1. National Health and Medical Research Council. *Recommendations for Minimising Radiological Hazards to Patients, 1985*. Australian Government Publishing Service, 1986.
2. Russell JGB. The rise and fall of the ten-day rule. *British Journal of Radiology* 1986; **59**:3–6.

3

Intravascular contrast media

Intravascular contrast media have many applications in imaging practice including: IVP, angiography, venography, and CT scanning. Other uses include myelography, arthrography, and sialography. Iodine is the element responsible for producing radiographic contrast. It has a high atomic number and so produces high attenuation of X-rays. Iodine compounds such as intravascular contrast media therefore appear white on conventional radiographs and on CT scans.

When considering morbidity and mortality of intravascular contrast media, two properties are important: *osmolality* and *ionicity*. The older compounds in use are hyperosmolar compared with serum and are ionic. The hyperosmolality of these compounds is responsible for many adverse effects. The older hyperosmolar compounds, when injected, produce an uncomfortable flushed feeling and are associated with a high incidence of nausea and vomiting.

The newer compounds are of lower osmolality and produce less toxic effects. In particular, the incidence of nausea and vomiting is markedly reduced and there is less nephrotoxicity, as well as a reduction in the rate of anaphylactoid reactions. When injected, the newer low-osmolality compounds produce a warm feeling and also a strange taste or smell. These effects are transitory, lasting no more than a couple of minutes. Most of the newer compounds are also nonionic and therefore safe for intrathecal injection. Ionic compounds must not be used for myelography.

The major (and probably only) drawback associated with the low osmolality contrast media is their increased cost.

The remainder of this chapter is devoted to the treatment of contrast media reactions and has been written by an anaesthetist colleague.

A. CONTRAST MEDIA REACTIONS

Andrew Russell

Immediate generalised reactions should really be classed as *anaphylactoid* as the aetiology is clearly not IgE mediated, though clinically these reactions are indistinguishable from anaphylaxis.

The postulated mechanisms for this type of reaction to intravascular contrast material include:

1. Direct histamine release from mast cells and basophils.
2. Complement activation.
3. Disruption of the vascular endothelium and consequent recruitment of other chemical mediators such as kinins.

Risk factors

1. Previous adverse reaction to contrast (10–30-fold).
2. Allergic history including asthma (4-fold).
3. Conventional high osmolar media > lower osmolar nonionic media.
4. Intravenous > intra-arterial > injection into body cavities (e.g. thecal sac, joints).
5. Anxious patient.
6. Patient on beta-blocker medication.
7. Fatal reactions more likely in elderly, debilitated patient.

Clinical features

(a) Minor reaction (5–8%):

* Rash, flushed.
* Rhinitis, cough.
* Mild urticaria, pruritis.
* Nausea, vomiting.

(b) Major reaction (0.1%):

* Commonest manifestion is cardiovascular collapse.
* Bronchospasm, pulmonary oedema.
* Angioedema, laryngeal oedema.
* Vomiting, gastrointestinal cramps.
* Death (0.01–0.04%)

Treatment

(a) Minor reaction:

* Cease administration of contrast.
* Reassure patient.
* Establish intravenous access.
* Oral or parenteral antihistamines.

(b) Major reaction:

There are three key points to remember:

(i) oxygen;
(ii) adrenaline;
(iii) fluids.

(c) Detailed protocol for severe reaction:

(i)   Call for help.
(ii) ABC:
* Secure airway and maintain oxygenation.
* Secure iv access with large-bore cannula (18-gauge minimum).
* If pulseless, commence external heart massage.
* Institute regular monitoring of the patient including oxygen saturation, blood pressure, pulse rate, ECG; and commence recording of observations and drugs given.
* Remember simple manoeuvres (e.g. Trendelenberg position for hypotension).
(iii) Adrenaline:
* The drug of choice, and should be used early; 3–5 ml of 1:10 000 iv and repeat as needed or commence infusion.
* 0.3–0.5 ml of 1:1000 s/c or imi if very early in course of reaction, no iv access, unmonitored cardiac patient due to risk of arrhythmias.
(iv) Fluids:
* May need 1–2 litres and colloid solutions more effective than crystalloid in severe cases.
(v)   Ensure regular reassessment of adequacy of resuscitation of patient and, once stable, continue observation in hospital for at least 12 hours as late deterioration may occur.
(iv) Follow-up – the nature of the reaction and the response to treatment should be accurately documented. The patient is given a letter and advised to wear a warning device (e.g. a Medi-alert bracelet) should future administration of contrast be necessary.

(d) Cardiovascular collapse:

* If BP remains low, central venous pressure measurement is helpful.
* Rarely, severe hypotension may not respond to adrenaline and may necessitate the use of other inotropes such as noradrenaline, dopamine.
* iv H2 blockers may also be helpful in the case of prolonged, profound hypotension.

(e) Bronchospasm:

- If severe, this is the most difficult feature to treat. Adrenaline is the drug of first choice.
- If inadequate response consider:
- (i) continuous nebulised and iv infusion of beta agonists;
- (ii) aminophylline if no response to above;
- (iii) steroids though response not immediate;
- (iv) intubation and IPPV may be necessary.

(f) Pulmonary oedema

- The oedema that occurs during anaphylaxis is a membrane type and is associated with a volume deficit.
- Treatment is PEEP and cautious fluid replacement with colloid *not* morphine and diuretics.

(g) Angioedema, laryngeal oedema

- Early intubation is the treatment of choice.
- Following the adminstration of adrenaline the oedema does not progress.
- An H1 antihistamine should be administered to prevent recurrence.

B. PREVENTION OF ALLERGIC REACTIONS IN HIGH-RISK PATIENTS

Does the patient really need contrast (document reason in chart)?

Advise patient of risk of exposure to contrast. Reduce likelihood of reaction:

1. Use nonionic, low-osmolality contrast.
2. Cease or replace beta-blocker medication if at all possible.
3. Use a pre-treatment regimen:
   - Pre-medicate, e.g. Temazepam 10–20 mg 1 h prior to procedure.
   - Prednisone 50 mg po 13,7, 1 h precontrast.
   - Diphenhydramine 50 mg imi or orally 1 h prior if emergency procedure.
   - Hydrocortisone 200 mg iv immediately and 4th hourly till procedure.
   - Diphenhydramine 50 mg imi 1 h precontrast.

Remember, these precautions will not prevent all reactions.

Ensure staff skilled in the treatment of severe reactions and the appropriate resuscitation equipment is immediately available.

Secure iv access with large-bore cannula and commence appropriate monitoring (blood pressure, ECG, oxygen saturation).

Document in the chart and on patient letter the response to contrast on *this* occasion.

Further Reading

1. Anderson JA. Allergic reactions to drugs and biological agents. *JAMA* 1992;**268**:2845–2857.
2. Bush WH, Swanson DP. Acute reactions to intravascular contrast media. *AJR* 1991;**157**:1153–1161.
3. Desforges JF. Anaphylaxis. *NEJM* 1991;**324**:1785–1790.
4. Fisher MM. Treating anaphylaxis with sympathomimetic drugs. *BMJ* 1992;**305**:1107–1108.
5. Fisher MM, Baldo BA. Acute anaphylactic reactions. *MJA* 1988;**149**:34–38.
6. Fisher MM, Raper RF. Respiratory complications and anaphylaxis. *Ballière's Clinical Anaesthesiology* 1993;**7**:390–398.
7. Greenberger PA, Patterson R. The prevention of immediate generalized reactions to radiocontrast media in high risk patients. *J Allergy Clinical Immunology* 1991;**87**:867–872.
8. Liberman P. Anaphylactoid reactions to radiocontrast material. *Ann. Allergy* 1991;**67**:91–97.
9. Yunginger JW. Anaphylaxis. *Ann. Allergy* 1992;**69**:87–93.

SECTION II
Plain-film interpretation

4
Chest X-ray

A. Projections performed
B. Technical assessment
C. Diagnostic assessment of the chest X-ray
D. Radiographic anatomy
E. Interpretation of chest X-rays
F. Summary of CXR appearances in common disorders

A. PROJECTIONS PERFORMED

A standard chest X-ray (CXR) examination consists of two projections, as follows.

I. PA erect

The patient stands with his/her anterior chest wall up against the X-ray film; the X-ray tube lies behind the patient such that X-rays pass through the patient in a postero-anterior (PA) direction.

(a) Reasons for performing the film PA:

- Accurate assessment of cardiac size due to minimal magnification.
- Scapulae able to be rotated out of the way.

(b) Reasons for performing the film erect:

- Physiological representation of blood vessels of mediastinum and lung; in the supine position mediastinal veins and upper lobe vessels may be distended leading to misinterpretation, e.g. over-diagnosis of widened mediastinum on supine chest X-ray.
- Gas passes upwards: pneumothorax is more easily diagnosed, as is free gas beneath the diaphragm.
- Fluid passes downwards, therefore pleural effusion is more easily diagnosed.

2. Lateral

(a) Reasons for performing a lateral chest X-ray:

- Further view of lungs, especially those areas obscured on the PA film, e.g. posterior segments of lower lobes, areas behind the hila, left lower lobe which lies behind the heart on the PA.
- Further assessment of cardiac configuration.
- Further anatomical localisation of lesions.
- More sensitive for pleural effusions.
- Good view of thoracic spine.

In general, I would advocate the use of two views, as above, in the assessment of most chest conditions. Exceptions where a PA film alone would suffice are:

- 'screening' in young people (e.g. for insurance or diving medicals);
- large-population screening programmes (e.g. for TB);
- follow-up of known conditions seen well on the PA (e.g. pneumonia following antibiotics, metastases following chemotherapy, pneumothorax following drainage).

(b) Other projections may be used as follows.

1. AP/supine X-ray

- Where the patient is too ill to stand (i.e. ICU, CCU, trauma, very elderly patients).
- Note that the mediastinum will appear wider on an AP supine film due to venous distension and magnification; this may lead to an incorrect diagnosis of widened mediastinum which may be a trap, e.g. in a chest trauma patient where aortic rupture needs to be excluded.

2. Expiratory film

- Suspected pneumothorax.
- Suspected bronchial obstruction with air trapping (e.g. inhaled foreign body in a child).

3. Decubitus film

- Radiograph performed with the patient lying on his/her side.
- Used occasionally in patients too ill to stand to exclude pleural effusion or pneumothorax.

4. Lordotic view

- Radiograph taken with the patient leaning backwards against the X-ray film and the X-ray tube is angled up.
- Shows the apical region which may be obscured by overlying ribs and clavicle on the PA film.
- Used less since the advent of CT.

5. Oblique views

- Used to show the ribs or sternum.

B. TECHNICAL ASSESSMENT

Prior to making diagnostic pronouncements, pause briefly to assess the technical quality of the PA film; the following factors should be considered.

1. Ensure patient properly centred on film

- The radiograph should include the lung apices and both costo-phrenic angles.
- Rotation: the easiest way to ensure that there is no rotation is to check that the spinous processes of the upper thoracic vertebrae lie midway between the medial ends of the clavicles.

2. Ensure adequate inspiration

- Diaphragms should lie at the level of the 5th or 6th ribs anteriorly.
- Straight trachea in children.

3. Ensure proper exposure

- The lower thoracic vertebral bodies should be faintly discernible through the heart.
- Blood vessels to the left lower lobe should be seen through the heart.
- Most dedicated departments use 'high kilovolt (kV)' techniques for chest radiography; this produces a less 'contrasty' film, i.e. the film looks more grey than black and white: the lungs and mediastinal outlines are shown superbly with this technique; and the ribs are less well visualised.

C. DIAGNOSTIC ASSESSMENT OF THE CHEST X-RAY

A teacher of mine once said that the best aid to viewing chest X-rays would be a 4 ft cage

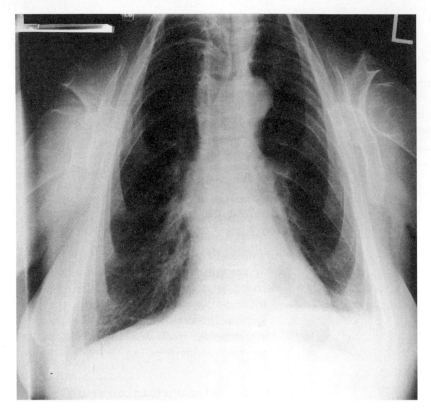

Fig. 4.1 Absent clavicles – cleidocranial dysplasia
This film illustrates the benefit of using a systematic approach in viewing radiographis. A gross finding such as absent clavicles can be suprisingly easy to miss. As such, this sort of case is a favourite with certain examiners.

strapped to the chest of the viewer! Most medical students to whom I show chest X-rays peer closely at the film, as if the answer is written in tiny letters on the patient's lungs.

The best tip I can give is to stand back a bit when viewing radiographs. If you don't believe me, try this small experiment: stand 3–4 ft away from a chest X-ray and assess it as directed below. Now move as close to the film as you like and see if any further information presents itself. In the majority of cases it won't.

When starting to look at radiographs try to use a system. This will help you avoid missing relevant findings. Below is the system I use. Try to incorporate the following.

1.   PA film

(a) Heart

- Position.
- Size.
- Configuration.

(b) Mediastinum

Identify normal structures:
- Trachea.
- Aorta.
- Pulmonary arteries.
- Superior vena cava (SVC).
- Azygos vein.

(c) Lungs

- Divide each lung into thirds, first from top to bottom, then from the hilum to the periphery.
- Look at top, middle, lower thirds, followed by medial, central, lateral thirds.
- Assess the vascular pattern: compare upper lobe vessels to lower lobe vessels.
- Look particularly at difficult areas where lesions are easily missed: behind heart; behind hila; behind diaphragms; lung apices.
- Check lung contours for signs of blurring or loss of definition: cardiac borders; mediastinal margins; diaphragms.

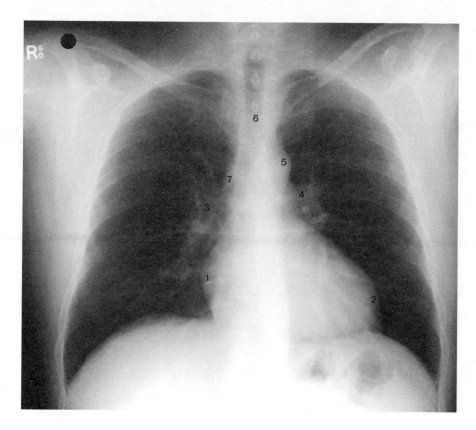

Fig. 4.2   Normal PA chest X-ray
Identity the following structures: 1) right heart border; 2) left heart border; 3) right hilum; 4) left hilum; 5) aortic knuckle; 6) trachea; 7) azygos vein.

(d) Bones

- Ribs.
- Clavicles (Fig. 4.1).
- Scapulae/humeri.
- Sternum on the lateral film.
- Thoracic vertebral bodies.

(e) Other

- In female patients check the breast shadows for evidence of previous mastectomy.
- Check below the diaphragm.
- Ensure stomach bubble in correct position.
- Check the axillae and lower neck for masses.

2.   Lateral film

(a)   Heart
- Size.
- Configuration.

(b) Mediastinum
- Identify the following: trachea; right and left pulmonary arteries.

(c) Lungs
- Retrosternal airspace.
- Retrocardiac airspace.
- Identify both hemidiaphragms.
- Posterior costo-phrenic angles: very small pleura effusions are seen with greater sensitivity than the PA film.

(d) Bones
- Sternum.
- Thoracic spine: lower thoracic vertebral bodies should appear blacker than upper ones; increased apparent density of the lower vertebral bodies may be the only sign of consolidation in the posterior basal segments of the lower lobes; this area is difficult to see on the PA film due to overlying diaphragm.

D. RADIOGRAPHIC ANATOMY

See *Figs 4.2 and 4.3*.

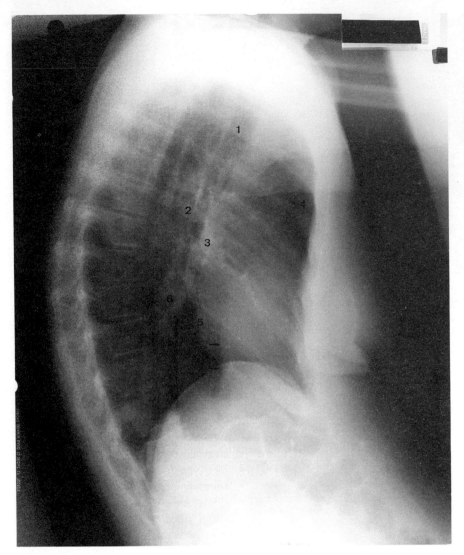

Fig. 4.3   Normal lateral chest X-ray
Identity the following structures: 1) trachea; 2) left pulmonary artery; 3) right pulmonary artery; 4) retrosternal airspace; 5) posterior heart border; 6) lower lobe arteries. Arrows point to the IVC.

E. INTERPRETATION OF CHEST X-RAYS

The lungs may be divided into two compartments: (a) the alveoli or airspaces; (b) the interstitium (i.e. soft tissues between the alveoli).

Disease processes may involve the alveoli or the interstitium, or both. One of the most important factors in interpreting chest X-rays is the ability to differentiate alveolar from interstitial shadowing.

I.   Alveolar processes

(a)   Signs of alveolar shadowing:

- Opacity tends to appear rapidly after the onset of symptoms.
- Fluffy, ill-defined areas of opacification.
- Areas of consolidation tend to coalesce.
- Two patterns of distribution tend to occur: segmental or lobar distribution and 'bats wing' distribution, i.e. bilateral opacification spreading from the hilar regions into the lungs with relative

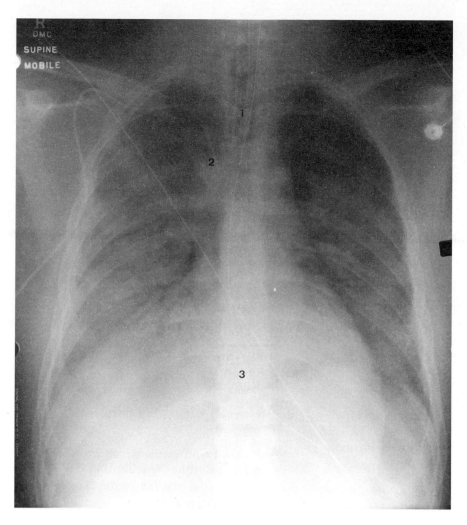

Fig. 4.4 Air bronchograms – pulmonary oedema
Air-filled bronchi are seen outlined by surrounding fluid-filled alveoli.
Note:
- endotracheal tube (1)
- central venous catheter (2)
- nasogastric tube (3)
- cardiac monitoring leads.

sparing of the peripheral lung fields, signifying extensive alveolar disease (e.g. pulmonary oedema).
- Air bronchograms (*Fig. 4.4*): air-filled bronchi are able to be seen as they are outlined by surrounding consolidated lung: air bronchograms are not seen in pleural or mediastinal processes.

(b) Causes of alveolar shadowing:

- Alveolar shadowing may be due to oedema fluid, inflammatory fluid, blood, or protein – they all have the same density on X-ray.
- Definite diagnosis may often be made where the CXR findings are correlated with the clinical signs and symptoms.
Common alveolar processes are listed below.

(c) Segmental/lobar alveolar pattern:

- Pneumonia.
- Segmental/lobar collapse.
- Pulmonary infarct.
- Alveolar cell carcinoma.
- Contusion (associated with rib fractures, pneumothorax, and other signs of trauma).

(d) 'Bat's wing pattern' (*Fig. 4.5*):

(i) Acute

Pulmonary oedema:
- cardiac failure;
- adult respiratory distress syndrome (ARDS);
- fluid overload;
- drownings and other causes of aspiration;

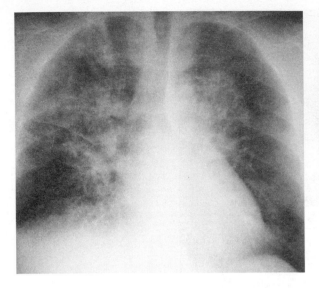

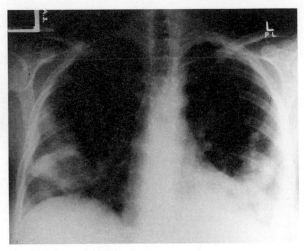

Fig. 4.6   Reversed 'bat's wing' consolidation –
lymphomatoid granulomatosis
Note predominantly peripheral distribution of consolidation
with relative sparing of the perihilar regions. This is a
typical distribution of changes in eosinophilic lung disease
for which there is a wide differential diagnosis.

Fig. 4.5   'Bat's wing' consolidation – pulmonary oedema
Bilateral perihilar consolidation with relative sparing of the
periphery.

- head injury or other causes of raised intracranial pressure;
- drugs and poisons (e.g. snake venom, heroin OD);
- hypoproteinaemia (e.g. liver disease);
- blood transfusion reaction.

Pneumonia:
- often 'unusual' etiology;
- pneumocystis carinii (AIDS);
- TB, viral pneumonias;
- mycoplasma.

Pulmonary haemorrhage:
- Goodpasture's syndrome;
- anticoagulants;
- bleeding diathesis: haemophilia, DIC;
- extensive contusion.

(ii) Chronic
- 'Atypical pneumonia': TB; fungi.
- Lymphoma/leukaemia..
- Sarcoidosis: interstitial form much more common.
- Pulmonary alveolar proteinosis.
- Alveolar cell carcinoma: localised form more common.

(e) 'Reversed bat's wing pattern'
(*Fig. 4.6*):

- Refers to processes which produce widespread alveolar opacification peripherally with relative sparing of the central zones.
- Loffler's syndrome.
- Eosinophilic pneumonias.
- Fat embolism: occurs 1–2 days following major trauma, particularly with fractures of the large bones of the lower limbs.

2.   Interstitial processes

Three types of pattern are seen in interstitial processes: linear, nodular, and honeycomb pattern. These may occur separately or together in the same patient, i.e. considerable overlap in appearances may be seen.

(a)   Linear pattern:

- Network of fine lines running through the lungs.
- Lines are due to thickened connective tissue septae and may be further classified as follows:

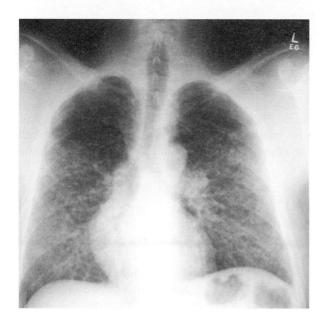

Fig. 4.7 Interstitial disease – sarcoidosis
Note numerous small, well-defined nodules with
associated

(i)   Kerley A lines: long, thin lines in the upper lobes
(ii) Kerley B lines: short, thin lines predominantly in the lower zones extending 1–2 cm horizontally inwards from the lung surface;
(iii) Kerley C lines: diffuse linear pattern through the entire lung.

(b) Nodular pattern (*Fig. 4.7*):

- Interstitial nodules are small (1–5 mm), well defined, and not associated with air bronchograms.
- Tend to be very numerous and distributed evenly through the lungs.

(c) Honeycomb pattern (*Fig. 4.8*):

- Represents the end-stage of many interstitial processes and implies extensive destruction of pulmonary tissue.
- Lung parenchyma replaced by cysts which range in size from tiny up to 2 cm diameter.

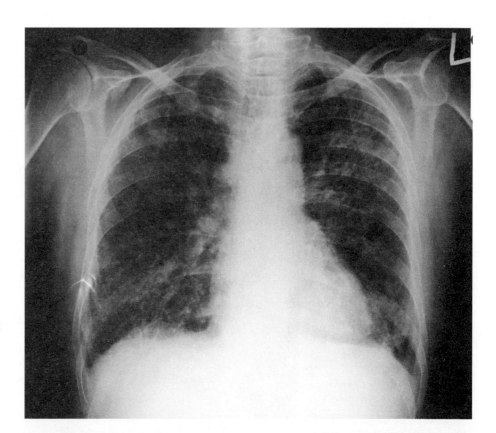

Fig. 4.8 Honeycomb lung
Note:
- loss of normal lung architecture
- coarse linear interstitial markings with small air-filled cystic spaces.

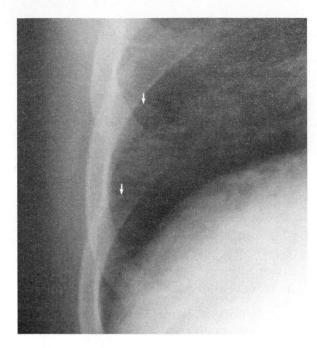

Fig. 4.9 Kerley B lines – interstitial oedema
Short, horizontal lines extending to the pleural surface
(arrows).

- Cysts have very thin walls>
- Normal pulmonary vasculature cannot be seen.
- Frequently complicated by pneumothorax.

The list of interstitial disease processes is extensive. Diseases may be roughly classified on the basis of whether they are acute or chronic or distribution in the lungs, i.e. upper or lower zones.

(i)   Acute

- Interstitial oedema.
  (a) Kerley B lines (*Fig. 4.9*);
  (b) associated with cardiac enlargement and pleural effusions;
  (c) may progress to, or be associated with, an alveolar pattern.
- Acute interstitial pneumonia – usually viral.

(ii)   Intermediate

- Lymphangitis carcinomatosa: prominent linear and nodular shadowing with Kerley

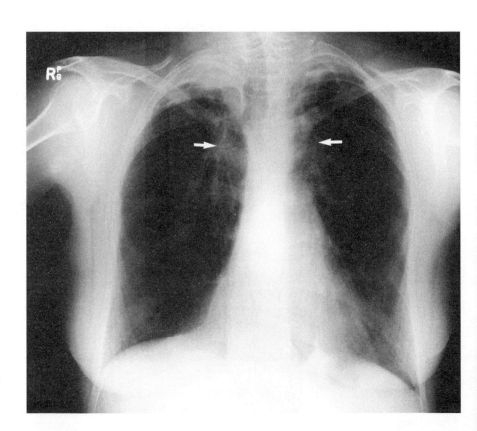

Fig. 4.10 Bilateral upper-zone fibrosis
Note loss of volume in both upper zones with elevation of both hila (arrows).
Differential diagnosis includes: TB, sarcoidosis, radiotherapy, and silicosis.

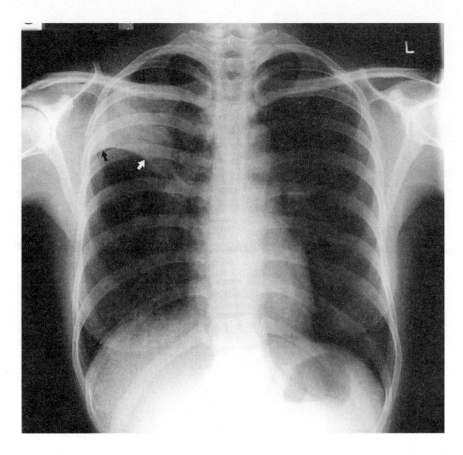

Fig. 4.11   Right upper-lobe consolidation
Note:
• opacity in the right upper lung with a well-defined lower margin (arrows) due to the horizontal fissure
• upward bowing of the horizontal fissure indicates some loss of volume in the right upper lobe.

B lines; often associated with mediastinal/hilar lymphadenopathy.

(iii) Chronic

Upper zones (Fig. 4.10)
• TB:
  (a) upper lobe fibrosis with loss of volume;
  (b) associated calcification in cavities;
  (c) acute miliary form gives a widespread fine nodular pattern.
• Sarcoidosis:
  (a) nodular form dominates;
  (b) often associated with hilar lymphadenopathy, though pulmonary involvement alone occurs in 25% of cases.
• Silicosis:
  (a) nodular and linear pattern;
  (b) associated with hilar lymph node calcification and enlargement;
  (c) may be associated with large confluent masses, i.e. progressive massive fibrosis (PMF).
• Extrinsic allergic alveolitis; bronchopulmonary aspergillosis; histiocytosis-X.
Lower zones:
• Fibrosing alveolitis.
• Asbestosis: may be associated with pleural plaques and calcification particularly of the diaphragmatic pleura.
• Rheumatoid disease:
  (a) associated with pleural effusions;
  (b) rheumatoid nodules.
• Other connective tissue disorders:
  (a) SLE;
  (b) systemic sclerosis;
  (c) dermatomyositis/polymyositis.
Honeycomb lung:
• End-stage of all diseases listed above.
• Also:
  (a) tuberous sclerosis;
  (b) amyloidosis;;
  (c) neurofibromatosis
  (d) cystic fibrosis.

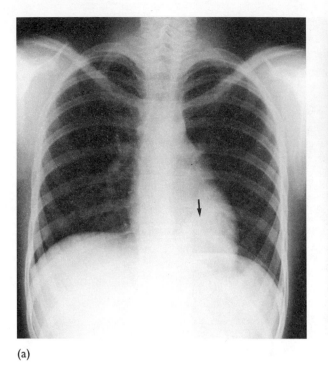

(a)

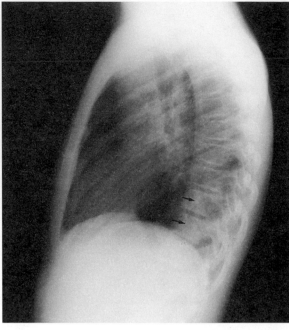

(b)

Fig. 4.12 Left lower lobe consolidation
a) PA film
Ill-defined opacity (arrow) seen through the left side of the heart.
b) Lateral film
Note increased apparent density of the lower thoracic vertebral bodies (arrows). This is an extremely important sign to recognize as lower lobe consolidation may be very difficult to see on the PA film.

3.   Localisation of lung lesions (*Figs 4.11–4.13*)

(a)   Silhouette sign:

Remember that in Chapter 1 it was stated that an object will be seen with conventional radiography if its borders lie beside tissue of different density. This especially applies in the chest where diaphragms, heart, and mediastinal outlines are well seen due to their lying adjacent to aerated lung.

Should a part of lung lying against any of these structures become non-aerated due to collapse, consolidation, or a mass, then the outline of that structure will no longer be seen. This is known as the 'silhouette' sign and is one of the most important principles in chest radiography.

Examples of the silhouette sign are listed below:

Part of lung that is non-aerated	Border that is obscured
Right middle lobe	Right heart border
Left lingula	Left heart border
Right lower lobe	Right diaphragm
Left lower lobe	Left diaphragm
	Descending aorta
Right upper lobe	Right border of ascending aorta
	Right mediastinal margin
Left upper lobe	Aortic knuckle *
	Upper left cardiac border

*Note that in severe collapse of the left upper lobe, the apical segment of the left lower lobe may be pulled upwards and forwards enough such that aerated lung lies beside the aortic knuckle: the aortic knuckle will therefore be seen in this situation.

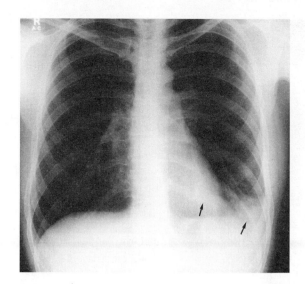

Fig. 4.13 Left lower lobe consolidation
A further case of left lower lobe consolidation showing an area of opacification in the left lower zone (arrows) obscuring the left diaphragm.

(b) Lung lesions adjacent to fissures:

Straight margins occur in the lungs at the pulmonary fissures. If an area of consolidation or collapse has a straight margin, that margin must abut a fissure and this can help in localisation, as below:

Right upper lobe
- Abuts horizontal fissure inferiorly on PA film;
- Abuts oblique fissure posteriorly on lateral film.

Right middle lobe
- Abuts horizontal fissure superiorly on PA film;
- Abuts oblique fissure posteriorly on lateral film.

Right lower lobe
- Abuts oblique fissure anteriorly on lateral film;
- Collapse causes rotation and visualisation of the oblique fissure on the PA film.

Left upper lobe
- Abuts oblique fissure posteriorly on lateral film.

Left lower lobe
- Abuts oblique fissure anteriorly on lateral film.
- Collapse causes rotation and visualisation of the oblique fissure on the PA film.

4. Patterns of pulmonary collapse (Figs 4.14 and 4.15)

Signs of lobar collapse are as follows.
- Decreased lung volume.
- Displacement of pulmonary fissures.
- Local increase in density due to non-aerated lung.
- Elevation of hemidiaphragm.
- Displacement of hila.
- Displacement of mediastinum.
- Compensatory overinflation of adjacent lobes.
Specific signs of lobar collapse:

(a) Right upper lobe: collapses upwards and anteriorly:

- Decreased volume of right lung.
- Elevation of horizontal fissure.
- Increased density of right upper zone.
- Loss of definition of right mediastinal margins.
- Elevation of right hilum.
- Tracheal deviation to the right.

(b) Right middle lobe:

- Increased density in right midzone with loss of definition of the right cardiac border.
- Lateral film: triangular opacity projected over the heart.

(c) Right lower lobe: collapses downwards and posteriorly:

- Decreased volume of right lung.
- Triangular opacity at the right base medially.
- Loss of definition of the right hemidiaphragm.
- Heart border not obscured.
- Elevation of right hemidiaphragm.
- Depression of right hilum.

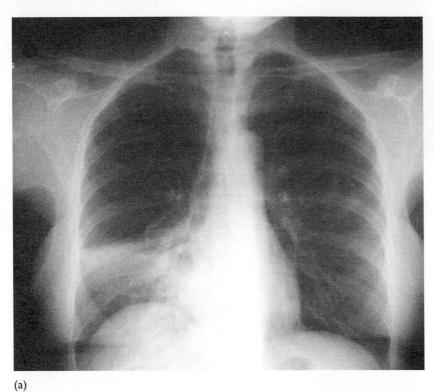

(a)

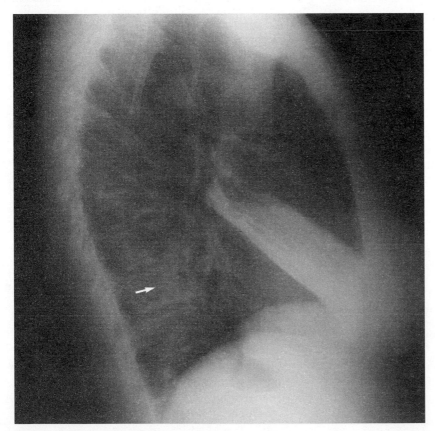

(b)

Fig. 4.14   Right middle lobe collapse

a) PA film

Note: • opacity in right mid- to lower lung
       • blurring of right heart border (compare with well-defined left heart border).

b) Lateral film

Note: • dense opacity projected over the heart
       • well-defined margins due to horizontal fissure anteriorly and oblique fissure posteriorly
       • consolidation is also seen posteriorly in the right lower lobe (arrow).

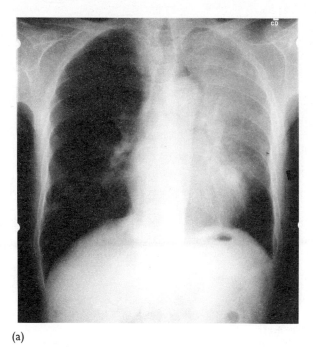

(a)

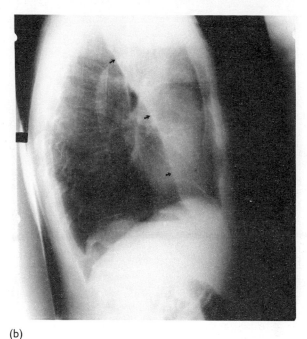

(b)

Fig. 4.15   Left upper lobe collapse
a) PA film
Note: • decreased volume of left lung
      • increased opacification of the left upper zone
      • loss of definition of left cardiac border and of left hilum.
b) Lateral film
Note: • large anterior opacity due to left upper lobe which has collapsed upwards and anteriorly
      • well-defined posterior margin (arrows) due to oblique fissure.

- Non-visualisation of the right lower lobe artery.
- Lateral film: increased apparent density of lower thoracic vertebral bodies.

(d) Left upper lobe: collapses upwards and anteriorly:

- Decreased volume of left lung.
- Increased density of left upper zone.
- Loss of definition of left upper cardiac border and left mediastinal margin; in severe left upper lobe collapse the aortic knuckle may be well outlined by elevated apical segment of the left lower lobe.
- Elevation of left hilum.
- Tracheal deviation to the left.
- Lateral film: increased opacity anteriorly which has a well-defined posterior margin due to the oblique fissure.

(e) Left lower lobe: collapses downwards and posteriorly:

- Decreased volume of left lung.
- Triangular opacity behind the left heart.
- Loss of definition of the left hemidiaphragm.
- Left heart border not obscured.
- Elevation of left hemidiaphragm.
- Depression of left hilum.
- Non-visualisation of left lower lobe artery.
- Lateral film: increased apparent density of lower thoracic vertebral bodies.

5.   Pulmonary vascular patterns

The normal lung vascular pattern has the following features:
- Arteries branching vertically to upper and lower lobes.

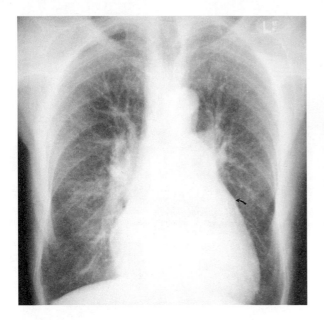

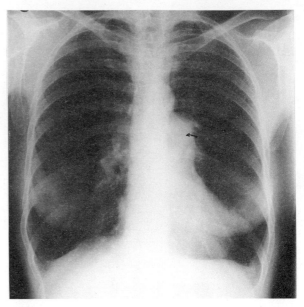

Fig. 4.16 Pulmonary venous hypertension – mitral valve disease
Upper lobe vessels are larger than those in the lobes, i.e. reversal of the normal pattern seen in the erect chest radiograph.
Note: • cardiomegaly
• prominent left auricle indicating left atrial enlargement (arrow)
• Kerley B lines.

• Veins running roughly horizontally towards the lower hila.
• Upper lobe vessels smaller than lower lobe vessels on erect CXR.
• Vessels difficult to see in the peripheral thirds of the lungs.

(a) **Pulmonary venous hypertension (*Fig. 4.16*):**

• Vessels in upper lobe larger than vessels in lower lobe on erect CXR.
• Associated with cardiac failure and mitral valve disease.
• Associated with pulmonary oedema and pleural effusion.

(b) **Pulmonary arterial hypertension (*Fig. 4.17*):**

• Pulmonary artery and its main left and

Fig. 4.17 Pulmonary arterial hypertension
Note: • prominent enlarged main pulmonary artery (arrow)
• rapid tapering in the calibre of more peripheral branches of the pulmonary artery.

right branches enlarged giving bilateral hilar enlargement.
• Rapid decrease in calibre of peripheral vessels ('pruning').
• Associated with long-standing pulmonary disease, e.g. emphysema, multiple recurrent pulmonary emboli, left to right shunts (VSD,ASD,PDA).

(c) **Pulmonary plethora:**

• Increased size and number of pulmonary vessels.
• Vessels seen in peripheral third of lung fields.
• Associated with left to right shunts (VSD, ASD, PDA).

(d) **Pulmonary oligaemia:**

• Decreased size and number of pulmonary vessels.
• Small main pulmonary arteries.
• General lucency (blackness) of lung fields.
• Associated with pulmonary stenosis/

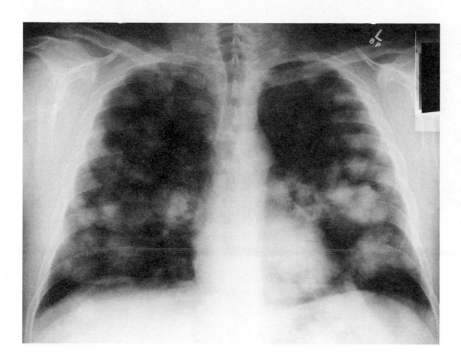

Fig. 4.18 Pulmonary metastases
Note multiple, well-defined masses throughout both lungs. Metastases tend to be more numerous peripherally due to haematogenous dissemination.

atresia, Fallot's tetralogy, tricuspid atresia, Ebstein's anomaly, severe emphysema.

6. Solitary pulmonary nodule

(a) Factors to assess:

- Size: greater than 4 cm. diameter highly suspicious of malignancy.
- Margin: ill-defined margin suggests malignancy.
- Cavitation: malignancy or infection.
- Calcification: rare in malignancy.
- Comparison with previous CXR to assess growth.

(b) Differential diagnosis:

- Bronchial carcinoma – suggested by evidence of rapid growth on serial CXRs, ill-defined margin, size greater than 4 cm.
- Solitary metastasis.
- Tuberculoma:
  (i)   calcification common;
  (ii) well-defined margin;
  (iii) usually 0.5–1.0 cm diameter;
  (iv) unchanged on serial CXRs.

- Bronchial adenoma:
  (i)   usually a carcinoid tumour;
  (ii) around 2 cm. diameter;
  (iii) calcification in one-third;
  (iv) hilar lymphadenopathy in 25%.
- Hamartoma:
  (i)   well-defined, lobulated margin;
  (ii) usually less than 4 cm diameter;
  (iii) calcification more common in larger lesions.
- Arterio-venous malformations – feeding vessels may be seen.

7. Multiple pulmonary nodules (Fig. 4.18).

(a) Metastases:

- Usually well-defined.
- Nodules of varying size.
- More common peripherally and in the lower lobes.
- Cavitation seen in squamous cell carcinomas, sarcomas, and metastases from colonic primaries.

(b) Abscesses:

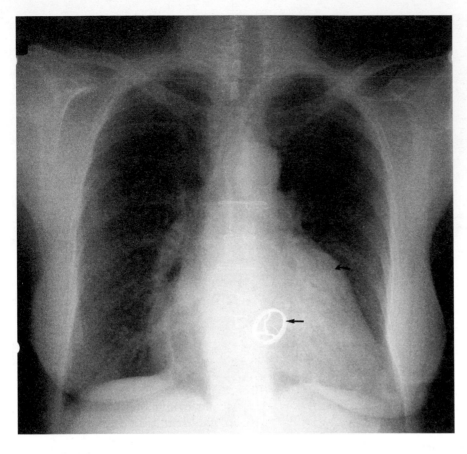

Fig. 4.19 Left arterial enlargement
Note:
- 'hump' on left upper cardiac border (curved arrow) due to prominence of the left auricle
- double edge to right cardiac border
- mitral valve prosthesis (straight arrow).

- Cavitation: thick, irregular wall.
- Usually Staphylococcus aureus.

(c) Hydatid cysts:

- Often quite large, i.e. 10.0 cm or more.

(d) Rheumatoid nodules

(e) Wegener's granulomatosis:

- Cavitation common.
- Associated paranasal sinus disease.

(f) Multiple arterio-venous malformations

8. Assessment of the heart

(a) Cardiac size:

- Cardiothoracic ratio is unreliable as a one-off assessment; of more significance is an increase in heart size on serial chest X-rays.
- Measurements may be used and are said to be more reliable than cardio-thoracic ratio.
- Maximum transverse diameter on PA film: 15.5 cm in male adults; 14.5 cm in female adults.

(b) Signs of specific chamber enlargement:

(i) Right atrium:
- Bulge of the right cardiac border.

(ii) Left atrium (*Fig. 4.19*):
- Convexity on the upper left cardiac border due to prominent left auricle.
- Double outline of the right cardiac border.
- Splayed carina.
- Bulge of the posterior heart border on the lateral film.

(i) Right ventricle:
- Elevated cardiac apex.

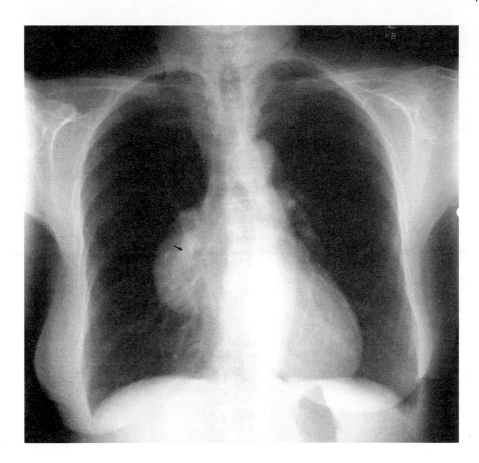

Fig. 4.20 Anterior mediastinal mass – Hodgkin's disease
Note:
- right-sided mediastinal mass
- right hilar structures can still be seen (arrow) indicating that the mass is either anterior or posterior
- loss of definition of the upper right cardiac border indicates that the mass is anterior.

- Bulging of the upper anterior heart border on the lateral film.
  (ii) Left ventricle:
- Bulging lower left cardiac border.
- Depressed cardiac apex.

9. Mediastinal masses

Signs of a mediastinal versus a pulmonary lesion:
- Sharp margin.
- Convex margin.
- Absence of air bronchograms.

Logical classification and differential diagnosis of mediastinal masses is based on localisation to the anterior, middle, or posterior mediastinum. In this regard, the silhouette sign and the lateral film are of most use.

(a) Anterior mediastinal masses:
- Merge with cardiac border.
- Hila can be seen through the mass.
- Masses passing upwards into the neck merge radiologically with the soft tissues of the neck and so are not seen above the clavicles (cervico-thoracic sign); a lesion seen above the clavicles must lie adjacent to aerated lung apices, i.e. posterior and within the thorax.

Differential diagnosis:

(i) Retrosternal goitre: cervico-thoracic sign, as above, i.e. mass not seen above the clavicles; displaced trachea.
(ii) Thymic tumour: may be associated with myasthenia gravis.
(iii) Thymic cyst.
(iv) Lymphadenopathy: Hodgkin's disease (*Fig. 4.20*); metastases.
(v) Aneurysm of ascending aorta.

(b) Middle mediastinal masses:
- Merge with hila and cardiac borders.

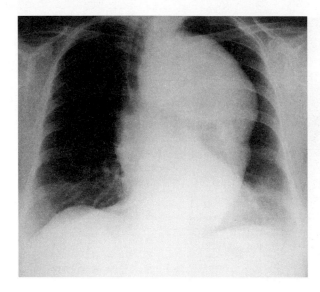

Fig. 4.21 Middle mediastinal mass – aortic aneurysm
There is a large aneurysm of the thoracic aorta causing displacement of the trachea.

Differential diagnosis:

(i) Lymphadenopathy: mediastinal/hilar; bronchial carcinoma, less commonly other tumours; lymphoma.
(ii) Bronchogenic cyst.
(iii) Aortic aneurysm (*Fig. 4.21*).

(c) Posterior mediastinal masses:

• Cardiac borders and hila clearly seen.
• Posterior descending aorta obscured.
• May be underlying vertebral changes.

Differential diagnosis:

(i) Hiatus hernia: located behind the heart; may contain a fluid level.
(ii) Neurogenic tumour: well-defined mass in the paravertebral region; erosion or destruction of vertebral bodies/posterior ribs.
(iii) Anterior thoracic meningocele: associated with neurofibromatosis.
(iv) Neurenteric cyst: associated with vertebral abnormalities.

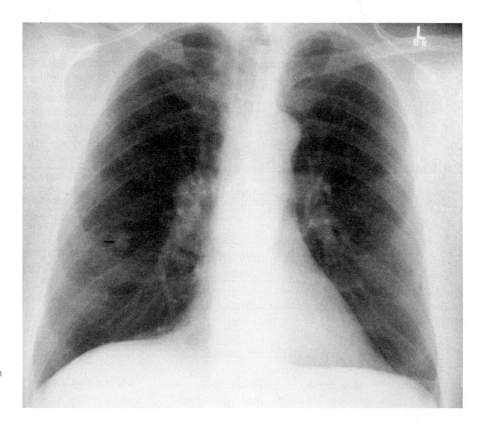

Fig. 4.22 Unilateral hilar enlargement – lymphadenopathy
Note:
• enlarged right hilar lymph nodes
• small primary carcinoma in the right lower lobe (arrow).

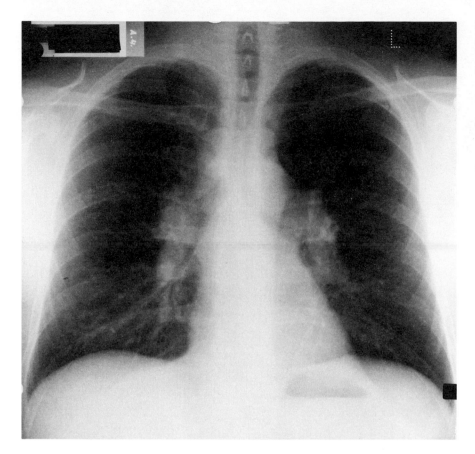

Fig. 4.23 Bilateral hilar enlargement – sarcoidosis There is increased size and density of both hila.

(v) Oesophageal duplication cyst.
(vi) Paravertebral lymphadenopathy.

10. Hilar disorders

Each hilar complex as seen on the PA and lateral chest radiographs comprises the proximal pulmonary arteries, bronchus, pulmonary veins, and lymph nodes. The lymph nodes are not visualised unless enlarged.

In assessing hilar enlargement, be it bilateral or unilateral, one must decide whether it is due to enlargement of the pulmonary arteries or some other cause like lymphadenopathy or a mass. If the branching pulmonary arteries are seen to converge towards an apparent mass, this is a good sign of enlarged main pulmonary artery (hilum convergence sign).

(a) Causes of unilateral hilar enlargement:

- Bronchial carcinoma (*Fig. 4.22*).
- Infective causes: TB; mycoplasma.

- Perihilar pneumonia: an area of pneumonia lying anterior or posterior to the hilum causing apparent enlargement on the PA film; is usually obvious on the lateral film.
- Other causes of lymphadenopathy (more commonly bilateral): lymphoma; sarcoidosis.
- Causes of enlargement of a single pulmonary artery: post-stenotic dilatation on the left side due to pulmonary stenosis; massive unilateral pulmonary embolus; pulmonary artery aneurysm (often calcified).

(b) Causes of bilateral hilar enlargement:

- Sarcoidosis (*Fig. 4.23*): symmetrical, lobulated, often associated with right paratracheal lymphadenopathy.
- Lymphoma: often asymmetrical.
- Metastatic malignancy: pulmonary/nonpulmonary primary (e.g. testes, breast).

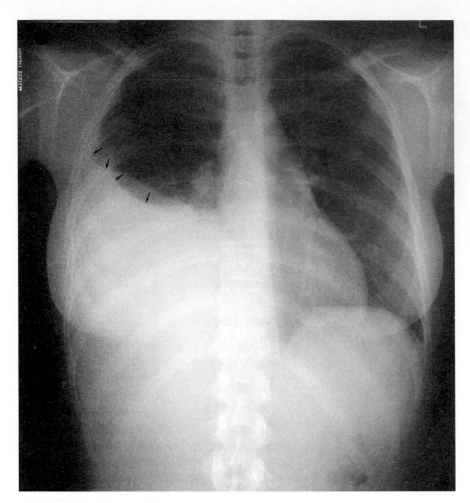

Fig. 4.24 Pleural effusion
Note:
- non-visualisation of right hemidiaphragm and costo-phrenic angle
- meniscus-shaped upper surface (arrows).

- Enlarged pulmonary arteries: pulmonary arterial hypertension.
- Silicosis: lymph nodes often calcified; associated with upper zone interstitial markings.
- Viral infection: infectious mononucleosis.

11. Pleural disorders

(a) Pleural fluid:

- Appearances not related to the nature of the fluid: transudate, exudate, blood, pus, lymph.
- Classical appearance of pleural effusion (*Fig.4.24*): homogeneous dense opacity; concave upper surface; meniscus, i.e. higher laterally than medially.

- Variants: loculations which may look like pleural masses; fluid in fissures; subpulmonic effusion: fluid trapped beneath the lung produces an opacity parallel to the diaphragm with a convex upper margin.
- Large effusions displace the mediastinum contralaterally.

Causes of pleural effusion:

- Cardiac failure: bilateral; right larger than left.
- Malignancy: bronchogenic carcinoma; metastatic.
- Infection: bacterial pneumonia; TB; mycoplasma; empyema; subphrenic abscess.
- Pulmonary embolus with infarct.
- Pancreatitis: usually left-sided.
- Trauma: associated with rib fractures.

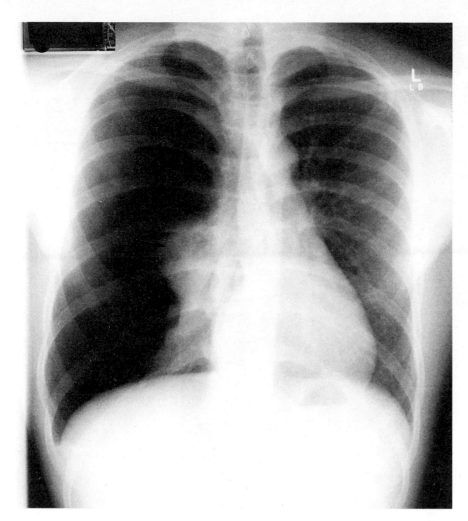

Fig. 4.25 Tension pneumothorax
Signs of tension pneumothorax as demonstrated in this case are as follows:
- total collapse of right lung (arrow)
- increased size of right hemithorax
- increased space between right ribs
- shift of the mediastinum to the left.

- Connective tissue disorders: rheumatoid arthritis; SLE.
- Liver failure.
- Renal failure.
- Meig's syndrome: associated with ovarian fibroma.

(b) Pneumothorax:

- Usually well-seen on a normal inspiratory PA film.
- Diagnosis of small pneumothorax easier on expiratory film.
- Lung edge outlined by air in the pleural space.
- Signs of tension pneumothorax:
  (i) distortion of lung;
  (ii) increased volume of hemithorax (displacement of mediastinum, depressed diaphragm, increased space between ribs) (*Fig. 4.25*).
- Pneumothorax in the supine patient (*Fig. 4.26*):
  (i) supine AP CXR may have to be performed in ICU patients or following severe trauma;
  (ii) pleural air lies antero-medially and beneath the lung so that the usual appearance as described for an erect PA film is not seen.
  (iii) mediastinal structures are sharply outlined by adjacent free pleural air: heart border, IVC, SVC;
  (iv) upper abdomen appears lucent due to overlying air;

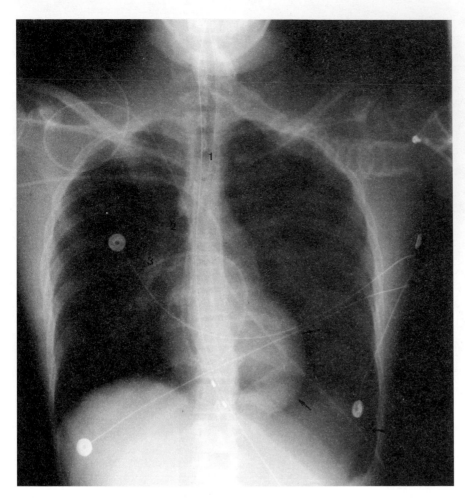

Fig. 4.26   Pneumothorax in a supine patient
Note:
- deep left costo-phrenic angle due to air beneath the lung (curved arrow)
- sharp definition of the left cardiac border due to air located anteriorly (straight arrows)
- endotracheal tube (1), with tip just above the carina
- central venous catheter tip in SVC (2)
- Swann Ganz catheter tip in right pulmonary artery (3).

   (v) deep lateral costo-phrenic angle;
  (vi) decubitus film with abnormal side up may be helpful.

Causes of pneumothorax:

- Spontaneous: tall, thin males; smokers.
- Iatrogenic: following percutaneous lung biopsy; ventilation; CVP line insertion.
- Trauma: associated with rib fractures.
- Emphysema.
- Malignancy: high incidence in osteogenic sarcoma metastases.
- Honeycomb lung.
- Cystic fibrosis.

(c) Pleural thickening:

- Secondary to trauma:
   (i) associated with healed rib fractures;
  (ii) dense layer of soft tissue, often calcified.
- Following empyema:
   (i) more common over the lung bases;
  (ii) often calcified.
- TB.
- Asbestos exposure:
   (i) irregular pleural thickening and pleural plaques.
  (ii) calcification common, especially of diaphragmatic surface of pleura;
 (iii) note that pleural disease is not asbestosis; the term asbestosis refers to the interstitial lung disease secondary to asbestos exposure.
- Mesothelioma:
   (i) diffuse or localised pleural mass;
  (ii) rib destruction uncommon;
 (iii) large pleural effusions common;

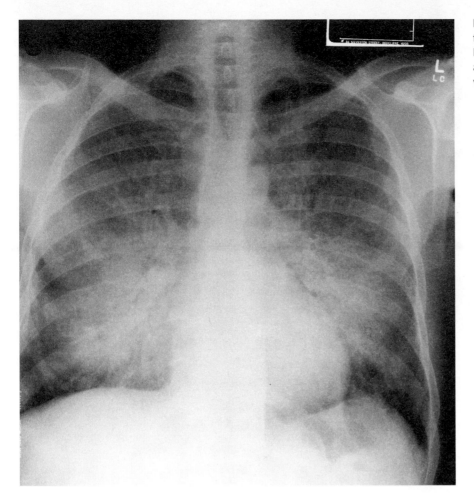

Fig. 4.27 Congestive cardiac failure
Note extensive bilateral alveolar shadowing in keeping with pulmonary oedema.

(iv) pleural plaques elsewhere in 50%.
- Pancoast tumour:
  (i) primary apical lung neoplasm;
  (ii) rib destruction with irregular pleural thickening.
- Pleural metastases – often obscured by associated pleural effusion.

F. SUMMARY OF CXR APPEARANCES IN COMMON DISORDERS

1. Cardiac failure (*Fig. 4.27*; see also *Figs 4.5, 4.9, 4.16,* and *4.19*)

- Cardiac enlargement.
- Pulmonary venous hypertension: upper lobe vessels larger than those in the lower lobe.
- Interstitial oedema:
  (a) Linear pattern;
  (b) Kerley B lines.
- Alveolar oedema: alveolar consolidation in 'bat's wing' distribution.
- Pleural effusions: right larger than left.

2. Emphysema (*Fig. 4.28*)

- Overexpanded lungs.
- Flat diaphragms lying below the 6th rib anteriorly.
- Increased retrosternal airspace on lateral film.
- Decreased vascular markings in lung fields.
- Increased antero-posterior diameter of the chest:
  (a) kyphosis;

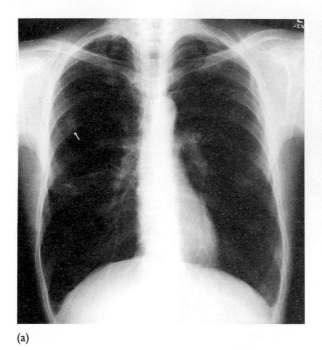

(a)

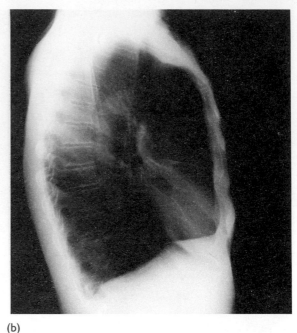

(b)

Fig. 4.28 Emphysema
a) PA film
Note: • overexpanded lungs
      • narrow mediastinum
      • healed fracture of right 7th rib: incidental finding (arrow)
b) Lateral film
Note: • flattened diaphragms
      • enlarged retrosternal airspace.

    (b) anterior bowing of the sternum.
• Bulla formation:
    (a) localised areas of decreased vascularity;
    (b) thin walls may be seen.
• Pulmonary arterial hypertension: prominent main pulmonary arteries.

3. Asthma

• Baseline changes:
    (a) overexpanded lungs;
    (b) thickening of bronchial walls, most marked in the parahilar regions.
• Complications:
    (a) lobar/segmental collapse due to mucous plugging;
    (b) pneumonia;
    (c) pneumothorax;
    (d) secondary aspergillosis.

4. Tuberculosis (TB)

• Primary TB:
    (a) usually asymptomatic;
    (b) healed pulmonary lesion may be seen – small peripheral nodule, often calcified; calcified hilar lymph node.
• Post-primary pulmonary TB (reactivation TB): predilection for apical and posterior segments of the upper lobes, plus the apical segments of the lower lobes:
    (a) variable appearances;
    (b) ill-defined areas of alveolar consolidation;
    (c) cavitation – thick-walled, irregular cavities; complicated by haemoptysis, aspergilloma, tuberculous empyema, broncho-pleural fistula;
    (d) fibrosis causing volume loss in the upper lobe;

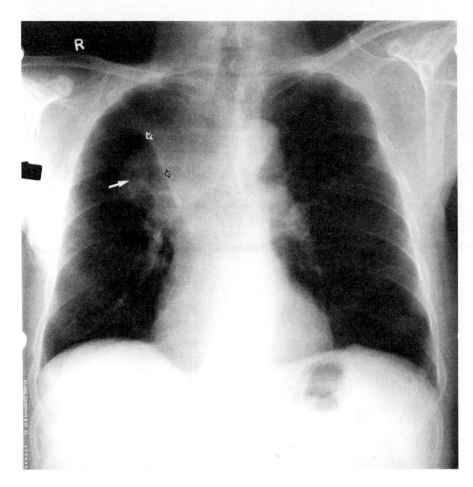

Fig. 4.29 Bronchogenic carcinoma

There is a large right hilar mass (white arrow) associated with collapse of the right lower lobe.

Note signs of right upper lobe collapse:

- decreased volume of right lung
- elevation of right hilum
- elevation of horizontal fissure (open arrows)
- non-visualisation of right upper mediastinal margin.

(e) calcification may occur with fibrosis;

(f) fibrosis and calcification usually indicate disease inactivity and healing, *but* one should never diagnose inactive TB on a single CXR: serial films are essential to prove inactivity.

- Miliary TB:
  (a) haematogenous dissemination which may occur at any time following primary infection;
  (b) tiny foci of approximately 2 mm diameter spread evenly through both lungs.

5. Bronchogenic carcinoma (*Figs. 4.29–4.31*)

- Wide range of appearances depending on stage at time of diagnosis.

- Pulmonary mass:
  (a) may be quite small: incidental finding;
  (b) mass greater than 4.0 cm diameter highly suspicious for malignancy;
  (c) cavitation, ill-defined margin;
  (d) calcification rare;
  (e) invasion of adjacent structures: mediastinum, chest wall.
- Segmental/lobar collapse.
- Persistent areas of consolidation.
- Hilar lymphadenopathy.
- Mediastinal lymphadenopathy.
- Pleural effusion.
- Metastases: lungs; bones.

6. Sarcoidosis (*Figs. 4.7, 4.10, and 4.23*)

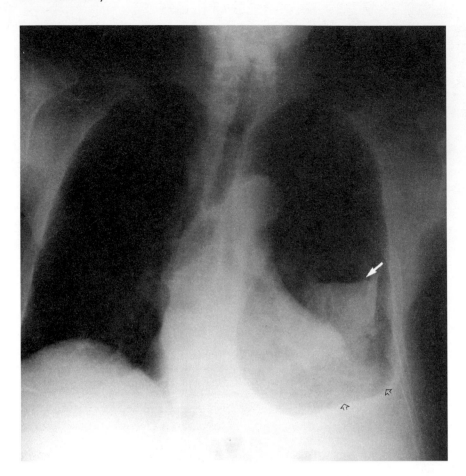

Fig. 4.30 Bronchogenic carcinoma
There is a cavitated mass (white arrow) in the left lower lobe associated with a left pleural effusion (open arrows).

- Hilar lymphadenopathy:
  (a) usually symmetrical and lobulated;
  (b) associated with right paratracheal lymphadenopathy.
- Interstitial lung disease:
  (a) multiple small nodules 2–5 mm diameter spread through both lungs;
  (b) predominantly in mid-zones.
- Rarely alveolar consolidation.
- Healing may lead to bilateral upper-zone fibrosis.
- CXR normal in 10% of cases.
- Lymphadenopathy alone in 50% of cases.
- Lymphadenopathy plus lung changes in 25% of cases.
- Lung changes alone in 15% of cases.

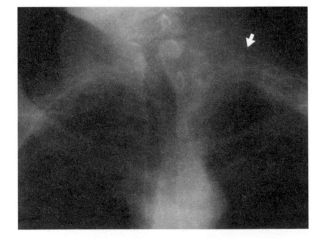

Fig. 4.31 Bronchogenic carcinoma – pancoast tumour
There is a left apical mass associated with destruction of the left 1st rib (arrow). Compare with normal right 1st rib.

7. Cystic fibrosis (*Fig. 4.32*)

- Bronchiectasis:
  (a) thickening of bronchial walls;

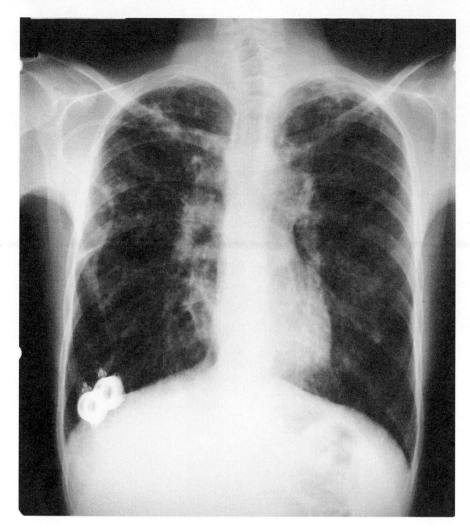

Fig. 4.32 Cystic fibrosis
Note:
- overexpanded lungs
- extensive linear densities and bronchial wall thickening
- central venous catheter.

(b) dilated bronchi.
- Overinflated lungs.
- Localised areas of collapse.
- Mucoid impaction in dilated bronchi: finger-like opacities.
- High incidence of pneumonia.
- Pulmonary arterial hypertension.

8. Interstitial pneumonia (fibrosing alveolitis)

- May see alveolar shadowing in the early stages of the disease.
- Interstitial linear and/or nodular pattern:
  (a) predominantly at lung bases;

  (b) irregular 'shaggy' heart border.
- Progressive loss of lung volume, particularly lower zones.
- Later honeycomb lung.

9. The post-operative chest X-ray (i.e. chest complications following non-thoracic surgery)

- Atelectasis: ranges from small areas of linear atelectasis to complete lobar collapse (*Fig. 4.33*).
- Pneumonia.
- Pleural fluid: may co-exist with basal collapse; unilateral pleural effusion may be seen associated with a subphrenic

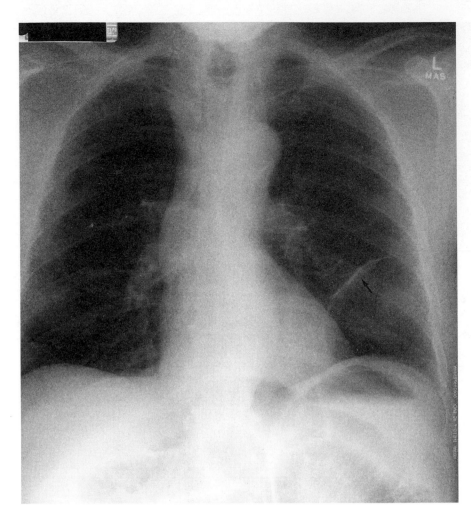

Fig. 4.33 Post-operative atelectasis
Typical appearance of an area of linear atelectasis (arrow) in the left lower lobe.

abscess.
- Cardiac failure.
- Pulmonary thrombo-embolism.

10. Chest X-ray following pneumonectomy

- Immediately post-pneumonectomy, the trachea is near the midline with a small amount of fluid in the pneumonectomy space.
- The fluid level rises over the following month with the trachea midline or pulled to the operative side.
- After two months, the pneumonectomy space is completely opacified due to fluid and/or fibrosis.

- Complications:
  - (a) empyema and broncho-pleural fistula: contralateral mediastinal shift; decrease in height of fluid level; appearance of air in a previously opacified pneumonectomy space;
  - (b) chylothorax: rapid opacification of the right hemithorax with shift of the mediastinum to the left;
  - (c) changes to contralateral lung: atelectasis; pneumonia; pulmonary oedema; pulmonary embolus.

11. Chest X-ray in chest trauma

- If possible, an erect CXR should be obtained.

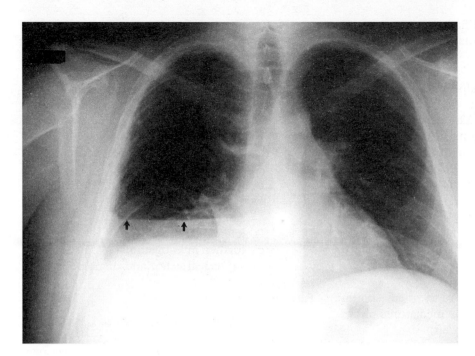

Fig. 4.34
Haemopneumothorax
Note the straight air-fluid
level (arrows) in the right
pleural space with no lateral
meniscus.

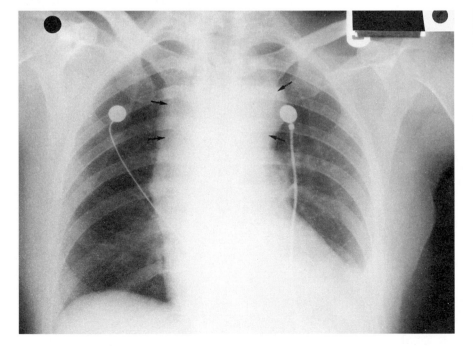

Fig. 4.35   Aortic rupture
Note:
- mediastinal widening
  (arrows) with non-
  visualisation of normal
  mediastinal structures due
  to haemotoma.
- non-visualisation of the left
  hemidiaphragm due to
  haemothorax.

- Rib fractures:
  (a) extensive views looking for subtle rib
      fractures are not advised in the acute
      situation, more important are associ-
      ated injuries;
  (b) fractured upper three ribs: suspect
      great vessel damage;
  (c) fractured lower three ribs: suspect
      upper abdominal injury (liver, spleen,
      kidneys);

(d) complications: flail segment, pneumo-
    thorax, subcutaneous air, haemo-
    thorax.
- Other fractures:
  (a) sternum: visualise on lateral view;
  (b) thoracic spine;
  (c) clavicle/scapula/humerus.
- Ruptured diaphragm:
  (a) herniation of abdominal structures
      into the chest;
  (b) contralateral mediastinal shift.
- Pneumothorax.
- Haemopneumothorax (*Fig. 4.34*): straight
  pleural fluid level without a meniscus.
- Pulmonary contusion: localised areas of
  alveolar shadowing.
- Pneumomediastinum:
  (a) vertical lucencies in the mediastinum;
  (b) air may outline the mediastinal pleura,
      especially on the left;
  (c) associated with subcutaneous air in
      the neck.

- Ruptured major airway:
  (a) severe pneumomediastinum;
  (b) pneumothorax.
- Aortic rupture – signs due to mediastinal
  and pleural bleeding (*Fig. 4.35*).
  (a) widened mediastinum which may be
      difficult to assess on supine film;
  (b) obscured aortic knuckle;
  (c) displacement of trachea and nasogas-
      tric tube to the right;
  (d) depression of left main bronchus;
  (e) associated fractures of upper three
      ribs;
  (f) left haemothorax;
  (g) further investigations – CT, transoe-
      sophageal echo, and angiography.

Further Reading

1. Felson B. *Chest Roentgenology*. Saunders, Philadelphia,
    1973.
2. Fraser RG, Pare JAP, Pare DP, Fraser RS, Genereux
    GP. *Diagnosis of Diseases of the Chest*, 3rd edn.
    Saunders, Philadelphia.

5
Abdomen X-ray

A. The standard abdominal series
B. Method of assessment of an abdominal X-ray
C. Common indications and findings

A. THE STANDARD ABDOMINAL SERIES

1. Supine antero-posterior (AP).

2. Erect AP

- Used to look for fluid levels and free gas.
- Therefore used for cases of possible intestinal obstruction or perforation.
- If the patient is too ill for the erect position, a decubitus film may be a useful substitute.

3. Erect chest

An erect chest X-ray should be a part of a routine abdominal series for the following reasons:
- Free gas beneath the diaphragms.
- Chest complications of abdominal conditions (e.g. pleural effusion in pancreatitis).
- Chest conditions presenting with abdominal pain (e.g. lower lobe pneumonia).

B. METHOD OF ASSESSMENT OF AN ABDOMINAL X-RAY (*Fig. 5.1*)

Due to a number of variable factors including body habitus, distribution of bowel gas and the size of individual organs, such as the liver, the 'normal' abdominal X-ray may show a wide range of appearances. For this reason, a methodical approach is important and the following check-list ('things to look for') should be used.

1. Hollow organs

- Stomach
- Small bowel: generally contains no visible gas, although a few non-dilated gas-filled loops may be seen in elderly patients as a normal finding.
- Large bowel
- Bladder: seen as a round, soft tissue 'mass' arising from the pelvic floor.

Fig. 5.1 a) and b) Normal abdomen
Identify the following features on the two radiographs: 1) liver; 2) right kidney; 3) left kidney; 4) spleen; 5) stomach. Black arrows: psoas margins; white arrows: properitoneal fat stripes; open arrows: bladder.

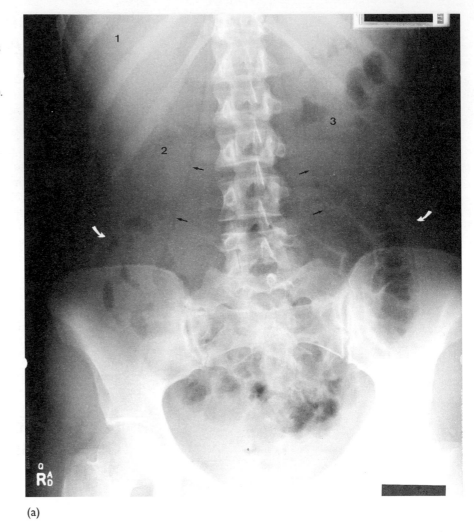

(a)

2. Solid organs

- liver.
- spleen.
- kidneys.
- uterus.

3. Margins

- diaphragm.
- psoas muscle outline (*Fig. 5.2*).
- flank stripe (properitoneal fat line).

4. Bones

- lower ribs.

- spine.
- pelvis, hips, and sacro-iliac joints.

5. Calcifications

- Aorta, other arteries: the splenic artery is often calcified in the elderly and is seen as tortuous calcification in the left upper abdomen.
- Phleboliths: small, round calcifications within pelvic veins; very common even in young patients and should not be confused with ureteric calculi.
- Lymph nodes: lymph node calcification may be due to previous infection and is common in the right iliac fossa and the pelvis.

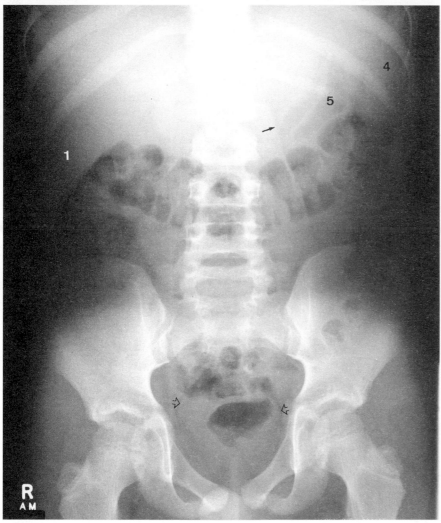

(b)

C. COMMON INDICATIONS AND FINDINGS

With the proliferation over the past two decades of imaging techniques, such as CT and ultrasound, and other modalities, such as endoscopy, the role of plain abdominal radiography has decreased. The abdominal X-ray is still a quite useful primary investigation in the patient with acute abdomen, depending on the specific presentation as outlined below. It is no longer recommended as a first-line investigation of abdominal masses, haematemesis, malaena, urinary tract infection, or vague abdominal pain. A number of less common indications will be encountered such as swallowed (or inserted) foreign body.

1. Bowel obstruction

- Distended loops of bowel with fluid levels on the erect view.
- Can distinguish small from large bowel obstruction.
- Small bowel loops have the following features: central location; several in number; relatively small (2.5–5.0 cm); small radius of curvature; valvulae conniventes (i.e. thin lines crossing the whole width of the bowel loop which are numerous and close together); no solid faecal content (*Fig. 5.3*).

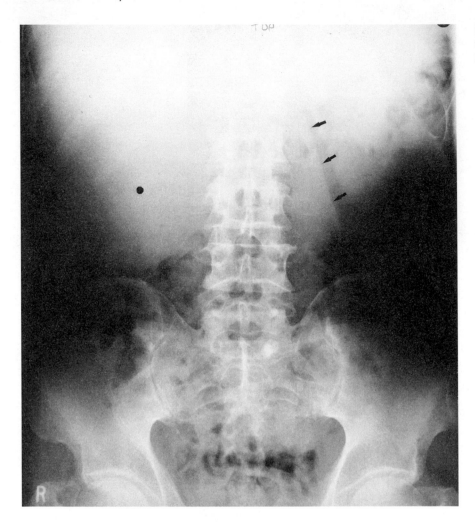

Fig. 5.2 Retroperitoneal mass – renal cell carcinoma
Note:
- normal left psoas margin (arrows); the left psoas muscle is outlined by retroperitoneal fat
- non-visualisation of the right psoas margin due to a large retroperitoneal mass (dot), in this case a renal cell carcinoma.

- Large bowel loops have the following features: peripheral location; few in number; relatively large (>5.0 cm); large radius of curvature; haustra (i.e. thick white lines which may or may not pass across the width of the bowel and are widely separated from each other); solid faecal content. (*Fig. 5.4*).
- Large bowel obstruction often has associated small bowel dilatation.
- Where there is plain film evidence of large bowel obstruction, a contrast enema may be helpful in showing the level and sometimes the cause.
- Mechanical obstruction may be difficult to distinguish from paralytic ileus.
- Paralytic ileus is of two types:
  (i) *Generalised*: refers to dilatation of small and large bowel loops with scattered,

irregular fluid levels on the erect view; may ocur post-operatively or with peritonitis.
  (ii) *Localised*: refers to dilatation of small bowel loops overlying a focal inflammatory condition; the dilated loops are referred to as *sentinel loops*: sentinel loops on the left occur with pancreatitis and left pyelonephritis; sentinel loops on the right occur with cholecystitis and right pyelonephritis.
- Occasionally a specific cause of intestinal obstruction may be identified on abdominal X-ray:
  (i) *Sigmoid volvulus*: massively dilated loop of sigmoid colon in the shape of an inverted 'U' which may pass upwards above T10; the limbs of the 'U'

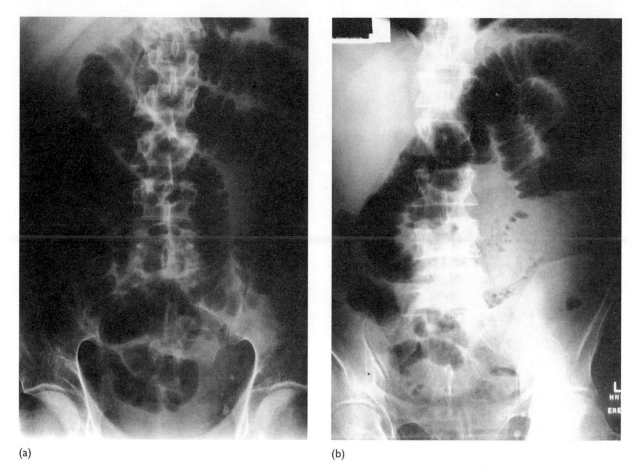

(a)   (b)

Fig. 5.3 Small bowel obstruction
a) Supine film
Note that small bowel loops are mainly central in position; numerous; measure less than 5.0 cm in diameter; have a small
radius of curvature; contain valvulae conniventes which pass across the bowel lumen; and are thin and close together.
b) Erect film
Note: • features of small bowel loops, as above
         • numerous air-fluid levels.

converge towards the left pelvis; the dilated loop contains no haustral markings and overlaps the dilated left descending colon (*Fig. 5.5*).

(ii) *Caecal volvulus*: markedly dilated caecum which may lie in the right iliac fossa or the left upper abdomen; the dilated loop usually contains one or two haustral markings; may see gas-filled appendix attached; collapse of the left colon; dilated small bowel (*Fig. 5.6*).

(iii) *Strangulated hernia*: gas-containing soft tissue mass in the inguinal region.

(iv) *Gallstone ileus*: small bowel obstruction; gas in the biliary tree; calcified gallstone occasionally seen lying in an abnormal position (*Fig. 5.7*).

2. Perforation

Perforation of the gastrointestinal tract can occur secondary to peptic ulceration, diverticular disease, malignancy, and ulcero-inflammatory conditions such as Crohn's disease and ulcerative colitis.

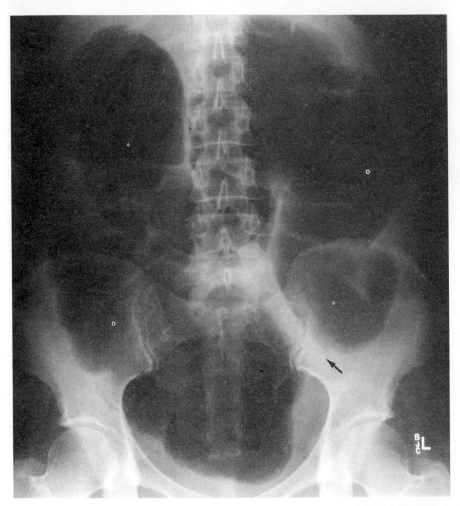

Fig. 5.4 Large bowel obstruction
The large bowel is dilated to the level of the sigmoid where there is an obstructing tumour (arrow).
Large bowel loops are peripheral in position; relatively few in number; have a wide radius of curvature; are greater than 5.0 cm in diameter; contain haustra which are thick and widely separated.
Compare and contrast the above features with those of small bowel obstruction demonstrated in Figure 5.3.

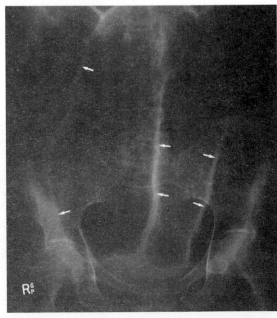

Fig. 5.5 Sigmoid volvulus
Note: • massively dilated sigmoid colon in the shape of an inverted 'U' rising to the level of T11
  • lack of haustral markings in the dilated loop
  • convergence into the pelvis of outer and inner walls of the dilated loop (arrows)
  • dilated proximal large bowel.

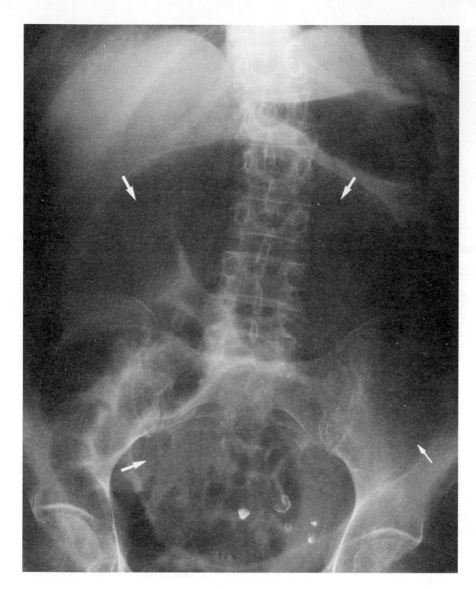

Fig. 5.6 Caecal volvulus
Note:
• massively dilated caecum lying centrally and to the left (arrows)
• dilated small bowel
• no dilatation of distal large bowel.

• *Erect chest X-ray*: free gas beneath the diaphragm.
• *Supine abdomen*: free gas outlines the bowel wall which appears as a thin white line; free gas may also outline the falciform ligament and the undersurface of the liver (*Fig. 5.8*).
• *Erect abdomen*: as little as 10 ml of free gas may be detected; decubitus films may be performed if the patient is too ill to stand.

3. Renal colic

Some 90–95% of renal stones are visible on plain films. In the context of renal colic, the abdomi-nal X-ray is usually performed as a prelude to IVP and thereafter for follow-up.

4. Other causes of acute abdomen

Plain films are generally unreliable in the diagnosis of the other causes of acute abdomen. All, some, or indeed, none of the signs listed may be seen in the clinical situations outlined below.

(a) Acute appendicitis

• Faecolith, i.e. calcific opacity in the right iliac fossa.

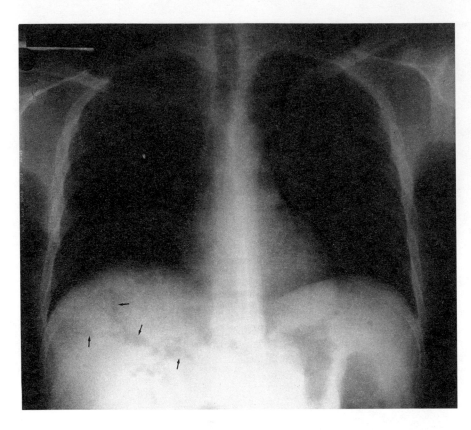

Fig. 5.7 Gas in the biliary tree
Note the branching gas pattern in the liver (arrows) conforming to the anatomy of the bile ducts. Differential diagnosis of this appearance includes:

- previous sphincterotomy or bile duct surgery
- fistula formation due to duodenal ulcer or malignancy of the biliary tree
- recent passage of a gallstone
- gallstone ileus
- patulous sphincter of Oddi in the elderly.

- Distal small bowel obstruction or localised paralytic ileus.
- Blurred right psoas margin.
- Lumbar scoliosis concave to the right.
- Gas in the appendix.
- Appendix abscess seen as a soft tissue mass in the right iliac fossa.

(b) Acute cholecystitis/biliary colic

- Soft tissue mass in the right upper abdomen.
- Overlying sentinel loops.
- Gallstones; only seen in 5–10% of cases.

(c) Pancreatitis

- Sentinel loops in the left upper abdomen, or generalised ileus.
- Loss of left psoas outline.
- Pancreatic calcification with chronic pancreatitis (i.e. calcification at about L1 passing up to the left in the line of the pancreas).

- Left lower lobe collapse and left pleural effusion.

(d) Acute colitis (*Fig. 5.9*)

- Bowel wall thickening or irregularity.
- Toxic megacolon; marked dilatation, often > 8.0 cm, usually of the transverse colon; often complicated by perforation.
- Gas in the bowel wall.
- Barium studies are contra-indicated in acute colitis.

(e) Abdominal trauma

- Free gas.
- Retroperitoneal fluid; loss of retroperitoneal fat planes (i.e. psoas margins and renal outlines).
- Bony lesions: fractures of lower ribs (commonly associated with hepatic, splenic, or renal damage), spinal fractures, pelvic fractures (commonly associated with bladder and urethral damage).

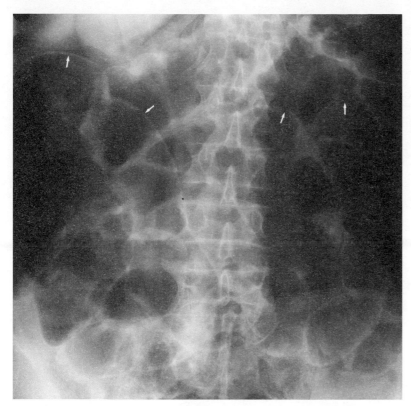

(a)

Fig. 5.8   Pneumoperitoneum
a) Supine abdomen
The bowel wall (arrows) is outlined by gas on both sides, i.e. gas within the lumen and free gas outside the bowel wall within the peritoneal cavity.
b) Erect chest
There is a large amount of free gas beneath the diaphragm.

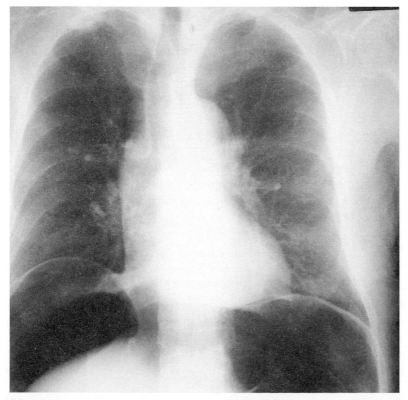

(b)

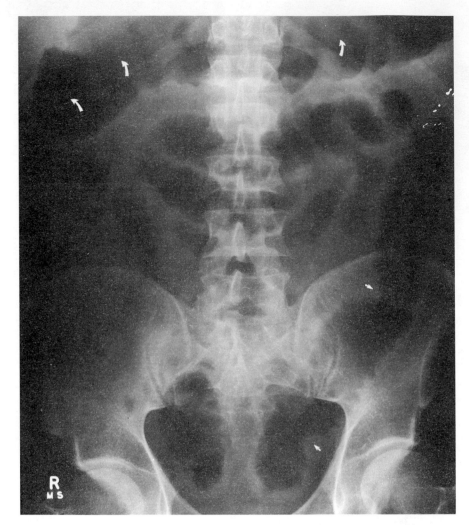

Fig. 5.9   Toxic megacolon
Note signs of acutely
inflamed large bo\
- loss of haust˜:˜ ˜nar˜ings
- irregular bowel wall with
  'thumb printing' indicating
  mucosal oedema (straight
  arrows).
Marked dilatation of the
transverse colon indicates
toxic megacolon (curved
arrows).

- Chest changes: pleural effusion, lower lobe collapse, ruptured diaphragm.
- Plain abdominal films are of limited use in assessing abdominal trauma; CT and ultrasound are more specific for the diagnosis of solid organ damage.

(f)   Abdominal abscess

- Mass, sometimes containing gas, and with a fluid level on the erect view.
- Displaced bowel loops.
- Localised or generalised ileus.
- Loss of adjacent margins (eg. psoas margin).

- Secondary chest changes; raised diaphragm, basal collapse, pleural effusion, subdiaphragmatic fluid level.

Further Reading

1. Paterson-Brown S, Vipond MN. Modern aids to clinical decision making in the acute abdomen. *British Journal of Surgery* 1990;**77**:13–18.
2. Skucas J, Sparato RF. *Radiology of the Acute Abdomen.* Churchill Livingstone, 1986.
3. Young WS. Further radiological observations in caecal volvulus. *Clinical Radiology* 1980;**31**:479–483.
4. Young WS, Engelbrecht HE, Stoker A. Plain film analysis in sigmoid volvulus. *Clinical Radiology* 1978;**29**:553–560.

6
Skull X-ray

A. Trauma
B. Involvement of the skull in general conditions
C. Other signs seen on skull X-ray
D. Facial trauma

A. TRAUMA

With the advent of CT scanning for the assessment of acute head trauma, the role of the skull X-ray has decreased. Patients with suspected brain injury or intracranial haematoma following head trauma should proceed straight to neurosurgical consultation and CT as the presence or otherwise of a skull fracture will not significantly influence management in the majority of these cases. Indications for skull X-ray in head trauma include:

- suspected penetration/foreign body;
- large scalp laceration/haematoma;
- suspected depressed skull fracture;
- CSF/blood from nose/ear;
- altered consciousness;
- focal CNS signs/symptoms.

It must be stressed, however, that CT is generally preferable for assessment of cranial trauma as skull X-ray cannot delineate brain damage or diagnose intracranial haemorrhage.

The following projections should be performed as a routine skull series for trauma:

1. *Lateral* – performed with the patient supine using a horizontal X-ray beam to demonstrate fluid levels.
2. *Antero-posterior (AP)* – to assess the frontal region.
3. *Towne's view* – to assess the occipital region.
4. *Lateral cervical spine* – should always be performed in major trauma.

1. Fractures

Fractures need to be differentiated from normal lucent linear markings in the skull (i.e. sutures and vascular markings).

(a) Sutures:

- Position; appearance.
- Sutures tend to be constant in position, so this is the most important parameter.
- *Lateral film*:
  (i) coronal sutures between frontal and parietal bones;
  (ii) lambdoid suture between parietal and occipital bones:
  (iii) may also see temporo-parietal and temporo-occipital sutures.

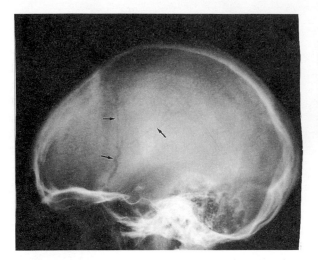

Fig. 6.1   Normal skull – vascular markings
The grooves formed by the middle meningeal vessels are well demonstrated (arrows). Note the typical features of vascular markings:
- tortuosity
- branching pattern
- distal tapering.

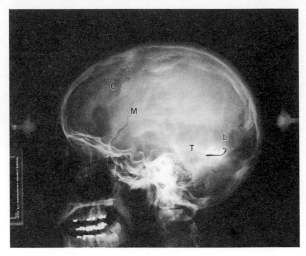

Fig. 6.2   Normal skull – vascular markings and sutures
Note:
- coronal suture (C)
- lambdoid suture (L)
- temporo-parietal suture (T)
- middle meningeal vessels (M)
- convolutional markings, i.e. normal impressions on the inner surface of the skull which tend to be more prominent in children.

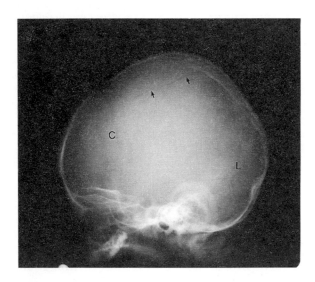

Fig. 6.3   Linear skull fracture
Note the typical features of a skull fracture (arrows):
- linear, non-branching
- able to be differentiated from the coronal (C) and lambdoid (L) sutures.

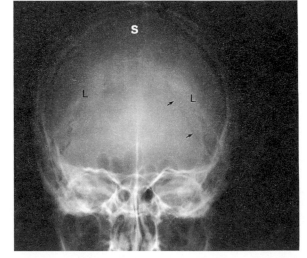

Fig. 6.4   Skull fractures
Towne's view to show the occipital bone.
Note:
- linear fracture (arrows) in the left occipital bone
- sagittal suture (S)
- lambdoid suture (L).

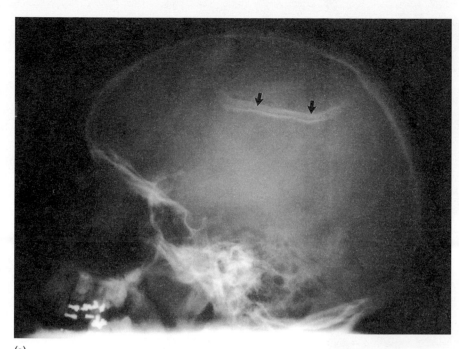

(a)

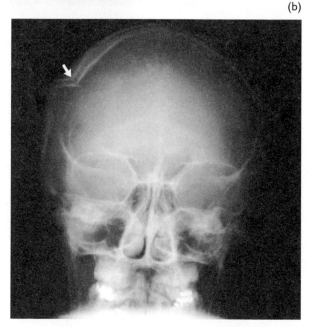

(b)

Fig. 6.5 Depressed skull fracture
a) Lateral view
The fracture is seen as a white band (arrows) due to overlapping bone fragments.
b) AP view
The configuration of the depressed fracture fragments (arrow) is well shown in this projection.

- *AP film*:
  (i) sagittal suture between parietal bones;
  (ii) lambdoid suture.
- *Towne's view*: lambdoid suture.
- Sutures may appear as straight or zigzag lines, or a combination of both.

(b) Vascular markings:

- Appearance; position.
- Vascular markings are made by venous channels and are quite variable in position, as such their appearance is the most important parameter.
- Vascular markings are tortuous and branching, have well-defined corticated (white) margins, become smaller as they pass upwards, and may cross sutures (*Figs. 6.1* and *6.2*).

Fractures have the following features:
- Linear.
- Non-corticated margin.
- Usually straight.
- Involve the full thickness of the skull vault and are therefore very lucent (i.e. black).

- Rarely cross sutures; the suture often separates if they do so (*Figs. 6.3* and *6.4*).
  The exception to the above is the depressed fracture which can be quite variable in appearance. A depressed fracture will often show as an irregular sclerotic area due to overlapping layers of bone. A tangential view is often helpful in showing the depressed fragment (*Fig. 6.5*).

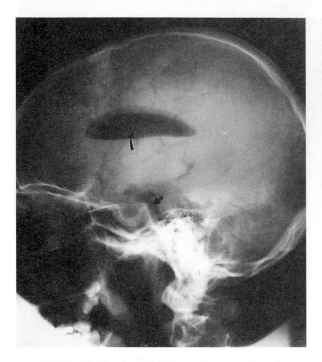

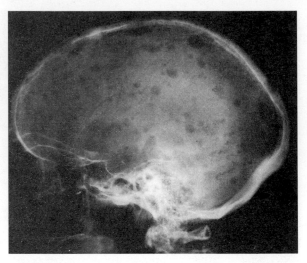

Fig. 6.7   Multiple myeloma
Multiple well-defined, 'punched out' lytic lesions. Metastatic carcinoma can also produce this appearance.

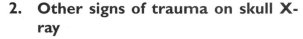

Fig. 6.6   Traumatic pneumocephalus
Air is seen in the basal cisterns (straight arrow) and lateral ventricles (curved arrow) following a base of skull fracture involving the sinuses.

2.   Other signs of trauma on skull X-ray

- Air in the cranial vault (*Fig. 6.6*).
- Air collection (aerocele) anterior to the frontal lobes.
- Air in the subarachnoid spaces and ventricles.
- Associated with penetration and fractures of the sinuses or petrous temporal bone.
- Fluid levels or complete opacification of sinuses.
- Pineal shift: although often quoted, this is an extremely unreliable sign. A large haematoma or severe cerebral damage may be present without midline shift.

B. INVOLVEMENT OF THE SKULL IN GENERAL CONDITIONS

I.   Metastases

- The vast majority are lytic regardless of the primary; sclerotic metastases are rare in the skull vault.
- The mandible is rarely involved.
- Irregular, destructive lesions.

2.   Multiple myeloma (*Fig. 6.7*)

- 'Punched-out', well-defined lytic lesions.
- May affect the mandible.

3.   Paget's disease

- In the active lytic phase seen as an area of lucency involving the lower frontal and occipital regions (i.e. osteoporosis circumscripta).
- Later seen as localised areas of sclerosis followed by generalised thickening of the skull vault.

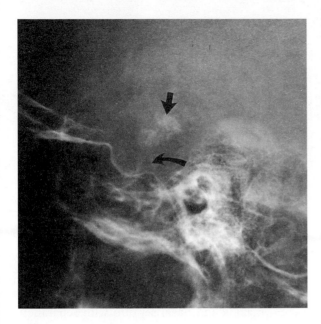

Fig. 6.8 Craniopharyngioma
Calcified suprasellar mass (straight arrow), with associated erosion of the dorsum sellae (curved arrow).

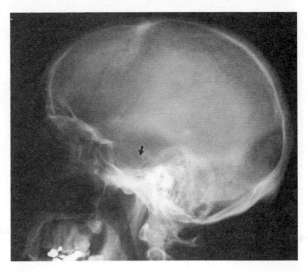

Fig. 6.9 Enlarged pituitary fossa
A pituitary adenoma is causing enlargement of the pituitary fossa with erosion of the dorsum sellae (arrow).

C. OTHER SIGNS SEEN ON SKULL X-RAY

Skull X-ray is not recommended as a first-line investigation for headache, raised intracranial pressure, epilepsy, psychiatric disorders, etc. The following signs, however, may be seen on skull X-rays performed for other reasons (or where other radiological tests are not available), and as such should be appreciated.

I. Calcification

Intracranial calcification may be due to a number of causes.

(a) Physiological (i.e. normal):

- Pineal.
- Choroid plexus.

(b) Tumours:

- Craniopharyngioma: 90% calcify in children; 40% in adults; calcification above the pituitary fossa (*Fig. 6.8*).

- Gliomas: 5–10% calcify, including 50% of oligodendrogliomas.
- Meningioma: 15% calcify and may be associated with hyperostosis (i.e. thickening of the skull vault adjacent to the tumour).

(c) Vascular lesions:

- Arteriovenous malformation.
- Large aneurysm.

(d) Infections:

- Toxoplasmosis, CMV, rubella: multiple peri-ventricular calcifications.

(e) Syndromes:

- Tuberous sclerosis: multiple calcified peri-ventricular nodules;
- Sturge-Weber syndrome: calcification of cortical gyri.

2. Enlarged pituitary fossa

(a) Normal dimensions:

Height – up to 11 mm; length – up to 16 mm.

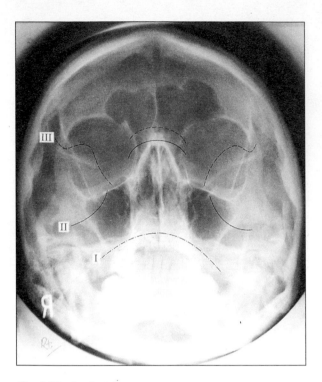

Fig. 6.10 Le Fort fractures.
A diagrammatic representation of the Le Fort classification of facial fractures.
Le Fort I —·—·—·—·—·—
Le Fort II ————————
Le Fort III ---------------

(b) Causes of enlargement:

- Para/intrasellar mass (e.g. pituitary adenoma, craniopharyngioma) (*Fig. 6.9*).
- Increased intracranial pressure.
- Empty sella syndrome: primary or secondary to treatment of pituitary lesions.

3. Generalised skull vault thickening

- Paget's disease.
- Long-term anti-convulsant therapy.
- Decreased intracranial pressure (e.g. ventricular shunt).

4. Signs of raised intracranial pressure

(a) Children:

Suture separation up to 8 years of age (wide sutures in children may also be due to infiltration by neuroblastoma or leukaemia), increased head size, erosion of the dorsum sellae.

(b) Adults:

Erosion of the dorsum sellae.

D. FACIAL TRAUMA

The facial bones are not well shown on normal skull X-rays. Specific facial views must be requested if facial fractures are suspected.

1. Maxillary fractures. (*Fig. 6.10*)

- The Le Fort classification is used to describe maxillary fractures.
- Le Fort I: fracture line through the lower maxilla and nasal septum with separation of the tooth-bearing portion of the maxilla.
- Le Fort II: fracture lines extend from the nasal bones in the midline through the medial and inferior walls of the orbits and the lateral walls of the maxillary sinuses, giving a large separate triangular fragment.
- Le Fort III: fracture lines run horizontally through the orbits and the zygomatic arches, causing complete separation of the facial bones from the cranium.

2. Zygomatic fractures (*Fig. 6.11*)

Fractures occur in 4 places:
- Orbital floor.
- Lateral wall of maxillary sinus.
  - Anterior end of zygomatic arch.
  - Lateral wall of orbit (i.e. diastasis of the zygomatico-frontal suture).

3. Blow-out fracture of the orbital floor (*Fig. 6.12*)

- Soft tissue mass in the shape of a tear-drop in the upper aspect of the maxillary sinus.
- Fracture seen in orbital floor.
- Air in the orbit.
- Herniation of orbital contents into the maxillary sinus well shown on coronal CT and MRI.

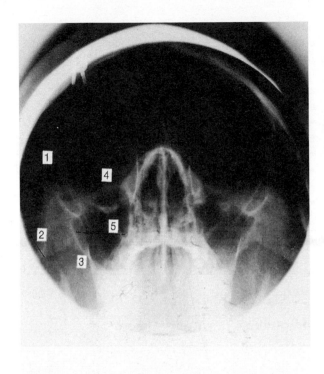

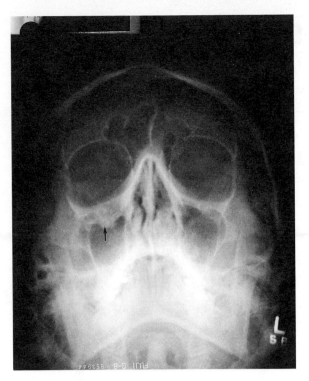

Fig. 6.11 Zygomatic fractures.
Diagrammatic representation of points to look for in suspected zygomatic fractures.
1. Diastasis of the zygomatico-frontal articulation in the lateral orbital wall.
2. Fracture of the anterior zygomatic arch.
3. Fracture of the lateral wall of the mazillary sinus.
4. Fracture of the orbital floor.
5. Fluid level in the maxillary sinus.

Fig. 6.12 Blow-out fracture of the orbital floor
Note depressed orbital floor with herniation of orbital contents (arrow) into the roof of the maxillary sinus.

4. Mandibular fractures

- Numerous views may be needed including local views of the temporo-mandibular joints and OPG (orthopantomogram) which gives a panoramic view of the tooth-bearing part of the mandible.
- Being 'U'-shaped, the mandible often fractures in two places.

5. Findings associated with facial fractures

- Fluid levels in the maxillary sinus.
- Soft tissue swelling.
- Air in the orbit or soft tissues.
- Orbital foreign bodies.

Further Reading

1. duBoulay GH. *Principles of X-Ray Diagnosis of the Skull*, 2nd edn. Butterworths, 1980.
2. Felson B. (ed.). The normal skull and its variations. *Seminars in Roentgenology* 1974;**9**(2).
3. Grainger RG, Allison DJ. Maxillofacial radiology: fractures (ch. 91). In *Diagnostic Radiology*. Churchill Livingstone, 1986.

SECTION III
Imaging techniques

7

Radiological procedures

A. Gastrointestinal tract (GIT) procedures
B. Genito-urinary tract procedures
C. Arteriography/angiography
D. Miscellaneous procedures

The following is a summary of the more commonly performed radiological procedures. *Interventional radiology*, which is rapidly becoming a sub-specialty in its own right, is covered in a separate chapter. Each procedure will be considered under the following headings:

- Indications.
- Patient preparation.
- Summary of method.
- Post-procedure care and precautions.
- Contra-indications.
- Complications.

A. GASTROINTESTINAL TRACT (GIT) PROCEDURES

1. Sialography (*Fig. 7.1*)

Indications:

- Suspected salivary duct calculus.
- Salivary gland swelling.

Patient preparation:

- Remove false teeth.

Method:

The mouth is rinsed with lemon or citric acid to promote flow of saliva and therefore make the

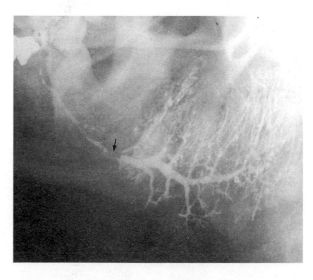

Fig. 7.1 Parotid sialogram – parotid duct calculus
Parotid duct calculus seen as a filling defect (arrow) in the contrast-filled parotid duct.

duct openings more visible. A fine cannula is then introduced into the duct opening and contrast-injected.

Post-procedure care:

- Nil specific.

Contra-indications:

- Allergy to intravenous contrast.
- Acute salivary gland infection.

Complications:

- Salivary gland infection (rare).

2. Barium swallow (i.e. examination of the oesophagus)

Indications:

- Dysphagia.
- Swallowing disorders in the elderly, following stroke or CNS trauma.
- Suspected gastro-oesophageal reflux.
- Post-oesophageal surgery.

Patient preparation:

- Nil by mouth for a couple of hours.

Method:

The patient is asked to swallow contrast material and films are taken. Barium is usually used, although for checking of surgical anastomoses, where leakage may be seen, a water-soluble material, such as Gastrografin, is preferable. Note that Gastrografin should not be used if pulmonary aspiration is suspected as it is highly osmolar and may induce pulmonary oedema if it enters the lungs. Images of the patient's oesophagus are recorded on cine-film, video, or X-ray film. Video is particularly useful in the assessment of swallowing disorders and these studies are often undertaken with the help and co-operation of a speech or swallowing therapist.

Post-procedure care:

- Physiotherapy and antibiotics if pulmonary aspiration has occurred.

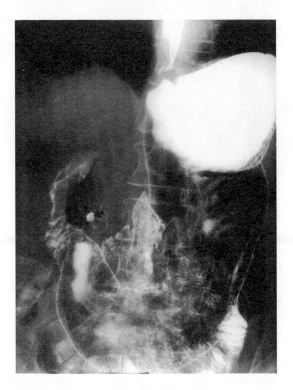

Fig. 7.2   Barium meal – duodenal ulcer
Double-contrast barium meal.
Duodenal ulcer (arrow) seen as a crater filled with barium. Note mucosal folds radiating from the ulcer.

Contra-indications:

- Known severe pulmonary aspiration.

Complications:

- Pulmonary aspiration.

3. Barium meal (i.e. examination of the stomach and duodenum) (*Fig. 7.2*)

Indications:

- Dyspepsia.
- Suspected upper GIT bleeding.
- Weight loss/anaemia of unknown cause. Assessment of anastomoses post-gastric surgery: use water-soluble contrast (e.g. Gastrografin).

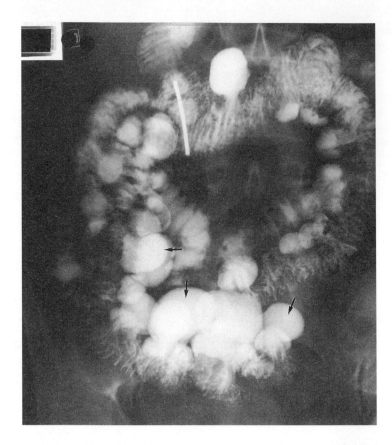

Fig. 7.3 Small bowel enema (enteroclysis) – jejunal diverticulosis
Excellent delineation of the small bowel. Note the filling of sac-like diverticulae (arrows) arising from the jejunum.

Patient preparation:

- Nil by mouth for 4–6 hours.
- No smoking on the day of examination.

Method:

This seems as good a place as any to introduce the concept of 'double contrast'. A single-contrast study is one where a hollow organ is filled with contrast material (e.g. barium). The outline of the organ can be appreciated, although not its mucosal surfaces (*Fig. 7.4*). If gas is then used to dilate the organ, the mucosal surfaces can be seen coated with barium. This is 'double contrast' (*Fig. 7.5*). The great majority of barium meals and enemas are performed in double contrast as it provides much better mucosal detail than single contrast. Single-contrast studies using barium only may be peformed in children, and occasionally in the very elderly.

In the case of a barium meal, the patient drinks a small amount of barium followed by gas-forming liquids and films are taken. An anti-

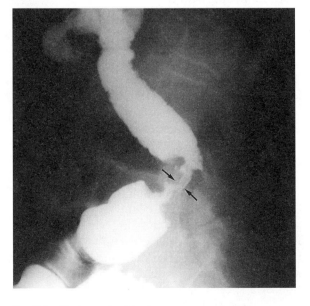

Fig. 7.4 Single-contrast barium enema – carcinoma
Constant area of narrowing with elevated margins giving the classical configuration of an 'apple core' shaped stricture typical of a carcinoma of the large bowel (arrows).

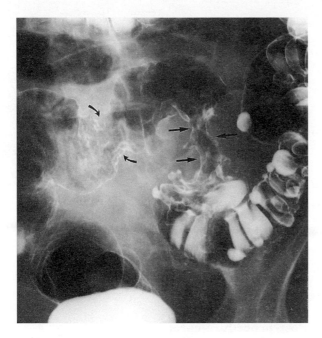

Fig. 7.5 Double-contrast barium enema – carcinoma
Note: • 'apple core' stricture (straight arrows)
• mucosal irregularity in the more distal colon indicating extensive involvement with carcinoma (curved arrows)
• diverticular disease of the more proximal colon.

spasmodic is commonly used to temporarily halt peristalsis and allow accurate imaging of the duodenum. Intravenous hyoscine is used. It rapidly halts peristalsis for 15–20 minutes. The side-effects are rare and due to anti-cholinergic effects (e.g. blurred vision, dry mouth). Hyoscine is contra-indicated in patients with cardiac ischaemia or glaucoma and intravenous Glucagon may be used in these cases.

Post-procedure care:

• Advise patient to drink plenty of water to aid the passage of barium from the bowel.

Contra-indications:

• Bowel obstruction.

Complications:

• Pulmonary aspiration.

4. Barium follow through (i.e. examination of the small bowel)

This is a simple procedure used to demonstrate and locate the site of a suspected partial small bowel obstruction. The patient drinks a quantity of barium and films are taken until the contrast either reaches an obstruction or enters the large bowel. Gastrografin should be used if there is any suspicion of a perforation.

5. Small bowel enema (*Fig. 7.3*)

Indications:

• Ulcero-inflammatory disease, especially Crohn's disease.
• Malabsorption syndromes.
• Miscellaneous small bowel conditions (e.g. tumour, Meckel's diverticulum).

Patient preparation:

• Nil by mouth on the day of examination, with a laxative on the evening before.

Method:

A nasogastric tube is passed in to the stomach and with the aid of a steering wire is then guided through the duodenum to the duodeno-jejunal flexure. A mixture of barium with either water or methyl cellulose introduced rapidly through the tube into the small bowel gives a double-contrast effect. Advantages of this technique over simple barium follow-through include:

• Better assessment of mucosal pattern.
• Much more rapid procedure.

The major disadvantage is the use of a nasogastric tube which is, of course, unpleasant to the patient.

Post-procedure care:

• The patient is warned of diarrhoea due to the large amount of fluid passed into the small bowel.

Contra-indications:

• Small bowel obstruction.

Complications:

- Problems with the nasogastric tube.

6. Barium enema (i.e. examination of the large bowel (*Figs.* 7.4 and 7.5)

Indications:

- Altered bowel habit.
- Lower GIT bleeding.
- Weight loss/anaemia of unknown cause.
- To outline and define a suspected obstruction (single contrast).
- Suspected perforation (Gastrografin).
- Check surgical anastomoses (Gastrografin).

Patient preparation:

Various bowel preparation regimes have been described, e.g. low-residue diet for 2–3 days, plus laxatives, with a bowel wash-out performed on the day of examination.

Method:

Barium is passed into the large bowel via a rectal cannula followed by air giving a double-contrast technique. Single-contrast technique may be used in the very elderly, or in children, or for suspected obstruction, as above.

Contra-indications:

- Toxic megacolon as may occur in ulcerative colitis.

Complications:

- Bowel perforation.
- Rare cases of allergy to the balloon used on the rectal catheter have been reported.
- Transient bacteraemia: patients with artificial heart valves should be covered by antibiotics.

7. Endoscopic retrograde cholangiopancreatography (ERCP)

Indications:

- Obstructive jaundice.

- Other biliary disorders (e.g. sclerosing cholangitis).
- Pancreatic disease (e.g. chronic pancreatitis).

Patient preparation:

- Nil by mouth for 4–6 hours.
- Mild sedation as for Endoscopy.
- Antibiotic cover.

Method:

The ampulla of Vater is identified and a small cannula passed into it under direct endoscopic visualisation. Contrast is then injected into the biliary and/or pancreatic ducts and films taken. Sphincterotomy, basket retrieval of stones, and stent placement may be performed at the time of ERCP.

Post-procedure care:

- Standard observations post-sedation.

Contra-indications:

- Acute pancreatitis.

Complications:

- Acute pancreatitis.

8. Percutaneous transhepatic cholangiography (PTC)

Indications:

- High biliary obstruction (i.e. at level of porta).
- Biliary obstruction not able to be outlined by ERCP.
- Precursor to stent placement for relief of biliary obstruction.

Patient preparation:

- Clotting studies.
- Sedation.
- Antibiotic cover.
- Nil by mouth 4–6 hours.

Method:

A needle is passed in to the liver and then slowly withdrawn as small amounts of contrast are injected. Once a bile duct is entered, contrast is more rapidly injected to outline the biliary system.

Post-procedure care:

- Standard observations of BP, pulse rate and temperature.

Contra-indications:

- Bleeding tendency.
- Biliary infection.

Complications:

- Haemorrhage.
- Septicaemia.
- Bile leak leading to biliary peritonitis.

---

9. CT arterial portography (CTAP)

Indications:

CTAP is used in the pre-operative assessment of patient with hepatic metastases being considered for partial hepatic resection. Standard CT with intravenous contrast is estimated to identify only 60% of hepatic metastases. CTAP identifies up to 95% of hepatic metastases, as well as providing more accurate segmental localisation and proximity to vascular structures.

Patient preparation:

- Cease anticoagulant therapy.
- Sedation occasionally used.

Method:

Via a femoral artery puncture selected angiography of the coeliac axis and superior mesenteric artery (SMA) is peformed. The catheter is then left in the SMA distal to the origin of any aberrant hepatic artery branches (seen in 25% of patients). The patient is then taken to CT. CT scans are performed during contrast infusion into the SMA. Contrast passes through the bowel and into the portal vein giving bright enhancement of normal liver tissue. Metastases, which are supplied exclusively by the hepatic artery and not the portal vein, are therefore seen as low-attenu-

ation non-enhancing lesions well outlined against the normally enhancing liver.

Post-procedure care, contra-indications, and complications:

- See following section on arteriography.

B. GENITO-URINARY TRACT PROCEDURES

1. Intravenous pyelogram (IVP)

Indications:

- Renal colic.
- Haematuria.
- For other conditions, such as prostatism, urinary tract infection, and renal cell carcinoma, IVP has been replaced by other imaging techniques, especially ultrasound, CT, and scintigraphy.

Patient preparation:

Some sort of bowel preparation is usually recommended: I feel that this has limited usefulness. Dehydration of the patient is no longer recommended. For patients at risk of contrast-medium reaction (i.e. previous reaction to contrast), severe allergic history, or asthmatics, oral steroid may be given prior to IVP.

Method:

Preliminary films are taken mainly to identify the kidneys and diagnose any area of renal tract calcification. This is particularly important in renal colic where a ureteric stone is being sought. Intravenous contrast is then injected. Films are taken to show the kidneys, the collecting systems, ureters, and bladder. When the kidneys are obscured by overlying bowel gas, tomography and/or oblique projections are used to outline the collecting system. This is especially important in patients with haematuria where a small TCC of the collecting system may be the cause. A post-micturition film confirms drainage of both ureters and emptying of the bladder.

Post-procedure care:

* Nil.

Contra-indications and complications:

* See Chapter 3 on contrast medium.

2. Retrograde pyelogram

Indications:

* To better delineate lesions of the upper renal tract identifed by other imaging studies (e.g. IVP).
* Haematuria, where other imaging studies are normal or equivocal.

Patient preparation:

* Standard pre-operative preparation.

Method:

This procedure is usually performed in conjunction with formal cystoscopy. The ureteric orifice is identified and a catheter passed into the ureter. Contrast is then injected via this catheter to outline the collecting system and ureter. It is my experience that better images are attained by performing the contrast injection in the X-ray department after the patient has left the recovery ward, rather than obtaining mobile films in theatre.

Post-procedure care:

* Standard post-operative care and observations.

Contra-indications:

* Urinary tract infection.

Complications:

* Rupture of ureter and collecting systems.

3. Ascending urethrogram

Indications:

* Prior to urethral catheterisation in any patient with an anterior pelvic fracture/dislo-

cation, or with blood at the uretheral meatus following trauma.
* Pre- and post-operative assessment of urethral stricture.
* Outline urethral anomalies (e.g. hypospadias).

Patient preparation:

* Nil.

Method:

A small catheter is passed into the distal urethra and contrast-injected. Films are obtained in the oblique projection. The posterior urethra is usually not opacified via the ascending method. Should this area need to be examined, a micturating cysto-urethrogram will be required.

Post-procedure care:

* Nil.

Contra-indications:

* Urinary tract infection.
* Recent urethral instrumentation.

Complications:

* Urethral trauma (rare).

4. Micturating cysto-urethrogram (MCU)

Indications:

* Urinary tract infection in children, i.e. for assessment of vesico-ureteric reflux.
* Suspected posterior urethral valves in male children.
* Posterior urethral problems in male adults.
* Stress incontinence in female adults.
* Post-prostatic surgery, i.e. to check anastomoses and the integrity of the bladder base.

Patient preparation:

* Antibiotic cover is often used.

Method:

The bladder is filled with contrast via a urethral catheter. The catheter is withdrawn and films are taken during micturition. The particular indication will dictate the type and number of films performed.

Post-procedure care:

- Nil.

Contra-indications:

- Acute urinary tract infection should not be present at the time of examination.

Complication:

- Urinary tract infection.
- Trauma due to catheterisation.

5. Hysterosalpingogram (HSG)

Indications:

- To check Fallopian tube status in infertility or following surgery.

Patient preparation:

- Nil.
- Sedation rarely used in nervous patients.

Method:

A speculum is inserted into the vagina and the cervix identified. The cervix is then cannulated and contrast injected. One or two films are then taken. Fallopian tube patency is indicated by spillage of contrast into the peritoneal cavity. Contrast is seen lying between small bowel loops. If no peritoneal spill can be seen, the examination may be repeated following the intravenous injection of Buscopan. This will relax the smooth muscle of the Fallopian tube wall and so exclude spasm as a cause of apparent obstruction.

Post-procedure care:

- The patient is warned to expect a small amount of vaginal discharge which may be blood-stained.

Contra-indications:

- Acute pelvic inflammatory disease.
- Pregnancy.

Complications:

- Infection.
- Allergic reaction to contrast (rare).

C. ARTERIOGRAPHY/ ANGIOGRAPHY

Some general comments on arteriography will be followed by notes on the common types of examination.

1. Digital subtraction angiography (DSA)

Digital subtraction is a process whereby a computer removes unwanted information from a radiographic image. It is particularly useful for angiography and the technique is referred to as DSA.

First, an image is taken of the relevant area prior to injection of contrast. This is called the 'mask'. Images are then taken with contrast in the blood vessels, and the computer then subtracts the 'mask' leaving an image of the contrast-filled blood vessels, unobscured by overlying bone, bowel, etc. (*Fig. 7.6*).

Patient preparation:

- Sedation may be required for nervous patients.
- Anaesthetic cover may be needed for children and for agitated patients, and where there is a high risk of contrast reaction.

Method:

The great majority of arteriography is done via a femoral artery puncture. Occasionally, if the femoral route cannot be used due to previous surgery or extreme tortuosity of the iliac arteries, the axillary or brachial arteries may be punctured. Catheter insertion is performed by the Seldinger technique as follows:

(a)

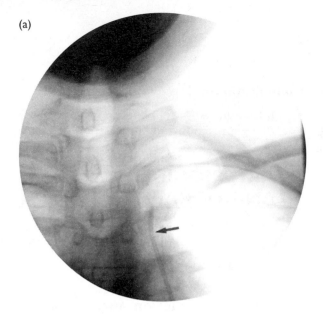

(b)

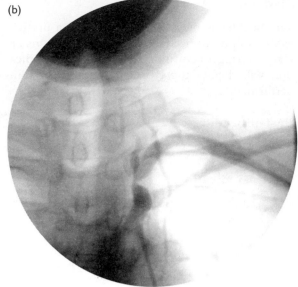

(c)

Fig. 7.6   Digital subtraction angiography
a) Mask flim
The mask film is taken immediately prior to injection of
contrast. Note: bone, soft tissue, arterial catheter (arrow).
b) Contrast film
Contrast is now seen in the left subclavian artery.
c) Subtracted image
The computer has subtracted the mask film from the
contrast film leaving an image of contrast-filled blood
vessels unobscured by overlying bone and soft tissue.
Note: tight, localised stenosis of the left subclavian artery
(arrow) proximal to the origin of the vertebral artery.

- The artery is punctured with a needle.
- A wire is threaded through the needle into the artery.
- The needle is removed leaving the wire in the artery.
- A catheter is inserted over the wire into the artery.

Depending on which artery is to be studied, variously shaped catheters are used. Indeed a bewildering array of catheters and wires has left few arteries in the body free from the prying eyes of radiologists.

Post-procedure care:

- Bed rest for several hours.
- Observe puncture site for bleeding/swelling and apply direct pressure if either of these is seen.

Complications:

(a) Due to contrast material.
   • See Chapter 3 on contrast material.
(b) Due to arterial puncture.
   • Haematoma at the puncture site.
   • False aneurysm formation.
   • Damage to brachial plexus with axillary artery puncture.
   • Arterial dissection.
   • Embolism due to dislodgement of atheromatous plaques.

It must be noted that newer techniques for examining arteries are being rapidly developed and accepted. These include ultrasound with Doppler, CT angiography (CTA), and magnetic resonance angiography (MRA). With the development of these techniques, the role of diagnostic arteriography will no doubt be reduced. The development of a vast array of interventional techniques, however, will ensure a steady increase in the therapeutic role of angiography, and these techniques are described in Chapter 8 on interventional radiology.

B. COMMON TYPES OF ANGIOGRAPHY

I. Cerebral angiography

Indications:

• Stroke/TIA.
• Investigation of subarachnoid haemorrhage, i.e. to outline aneurysm or other causes like arterio-venous malformation (AVM).
• Pre-therapy for AVM or carotico-cavernous fistula.
• Rarely for further characterisation of a mass or other abnormality seen on CT/MRI.

Complications:

• General complications of angiography.
• Cerebral embolism causing stroke (approx 0.3% overall).

2. Peripheral angiography

Indications:

• Symptoms of peripheral vascular disease, most commonly claudication.
• Trauma where arterial damage is suspected.

3. Renal angiography

Indications:

• Assessment of renal artery stenosis.
• Rarely for assessment of AVM or renal tumour.

4. Coelic axis/mesenteric angiography

Indications:

• GIT bleeding.
• GIT ischaemia.
• Pre-operative demonstration of vascular supply of liver tumour (i.e. surgical 'road map').
• CT arterial portography (see above).

5. Pulmonary angiography

Indications:

• Used in the diagnosis of pulmonary embolism where the ventilation/perfusion nuclear medicine study is equivocal.

Complications:

• General complications of angiography.
• Cardiac arrhythmias.

6. Coronary angiography

Indications:

• Ischaemic heart disease.
• Pre- and post-angioplasty assessment.
• Post-coronary artery bypass graft assessment.

Complications:

- General complications of angiography.
- Myocardial infarct.
- Arrhythmias.

D. MISCELLANEOUS PROCEDURES

I. Venography

Indications:

- Suspected deep vein thrombosis (DVT).
- Assessment of varicose veins.
- Assessment of venous strictures or narrowing due to external pressure (e.g. by tumour).
- Selective venography for various endocrine disorders.

Note: Venography of the lower limb has been largely supplanted by Doppler ultrasound. Ultrasound, however, has certain limitations: (a) the calf veins are imaged with difficulty; and (b) the pelvic veins are imaged with difficulty. Many clinicians don't consider thrombosis limited to the calf veins important as it is felt that pulmonary embolism from these veins is rare. Other clinicians feel that calf vein thrombosis can certainly propagate over time to involve the larger, more proximal veins and that it is therefore important to diagnose calf thrombosis: to say the least, this point is controversial. The difficulty with the pelvic veins is of more concern. Certainly, thrombus localised to the pelvic veins with normal femoral and popliteal veins is uncommon. It does, however, occur, and for this reason alone, I would advocate the use of venography in any case where there is remaining clinical suspicion of a DVT following normal Doppler examination of the femoral and popliteal veins.

Patient preparation:

- Nil.

Method:

A vein in the dorsum of the foot is cannulated with a butterfly needle and contrast injected. For venography of the upper limb the median cubital vein in the elbow is injected. The deep veins of the lower limb should be opacified up to the lower IVC. DVT shows in two ways: (a) filling defects in the deep veins; and (b) non-filling of the deep veins due to total occlusion with thrombus.

2. Arthrography

Knee arthrography was until recently the most common arthrographic procedure. It has been replaced by MRI and arthroscopy. The two regions most commonly examined with arthrography are the shoulder and wrist. Other joints rarely examined include the ankle, hip, and temporo-mandibular joint.

(a) Shoulder

Indications:

- Rotator cuff tear.
- Instability, i.e. recurrent dislocation: CT following arthrography is needed in the assessment of this problem.
- Adhesive capsulitis.

Patient preparation:

- Nil.

Method:

Following infiltration of local anaesthetic, a needle is passed into the shoulder joint using either an anterior or posterior approach. A double-contrast technique is used, i.e. water-soluble contrast plus air to distend the joint. Plain films are then obtained usually followed by CT.

Post-procedure care:

- The patient is warned that the joint may be painful for a day or two and is advised to avoid heavy exercise.

Contra-indications:

- Nil.

Complications:

- Septic arthritis.
- Chemical synovitis.

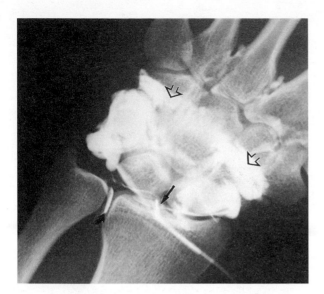

Fig. 7.7 Wrist arthrogram

Note: • needle in the radio-carpal joint (straight arrow)
• abnormal filling of the radio-ulnar joint space (curved arrow) through a defect in the triangular fibro-cartilage complex
• contrast in the midcarpal joint from prior injection (open arrows).

(b) Wrist (*Fig. 7.7*)

Indications:

Used following trauma to demonstrate the integrity of intra-articular and para-articular ligaments, most commonly the triangular fibro-cartilage complex though also the scapho-lunate and lunate-triquetral ligaments.

Patient preparation:

• Nil.

Method:

The mid-carpal joint is first injected with contrast to demonstrate any abnormal communications with the radio-carpal joint. The radio-carpal joint is then injected. Rupture of the triangular fibro-cartilage complex is diagnosed by visualisation of contrast entering the distal radio-ulnar joint.

Post-procedure care:

• The patient is advised to avoid exercise of the wrist for a couple of days.

Contra-indications:

• Nil.

Complications:

• Septic arthritis.
• Chemical synovitis.

---

3. Myelography

Indications:

For the assessment of spinal disorders myelography has been largely supplanted by CT and MRI. MRI is now the imaging method of choice for virtually all types of spinal disorder. Myelography is still quite widely practised, however, and is therefore included in this chapter.

Method:

A lumbar puncture is performed at L2/L3 or L3/L4 and a small amount of CSF aspirated. Water-soluble non-ionic contrast is then injected into the subarachnoid space and films are obtained of areas of interest, often followed by CT.

Post-procedure care:

• Bed rest is recommended for up to 8 hours followed by gentle mobilisation.
• High fluid intake to ensure adequate hydration is encouraged.

Contraindications:

• Previous reaction to intrathecal contrast.

Complications:

• Headaches: these are usually transient; however, if severe and persistent, may indicate an ongoing CSF leak from the puncture site necessitating a 'blood patch', i.e. a small amount of the patient's blood injected into the epidural space at the puncture site.
• Nausea and vomiting.
• Convulsions: very rare with the newer contrast media.

Further Reading

1. Hunt   RB,   Siegler   AM.   *Hysterosalpingography: Techniques and Interpretation.* Year Book Medical Publishers, 1990.
2. Krysiewicz S. Infertility in women: diagnostic evaluation with hysterosalpingography and other imaging techniques. *AJR* 1992;**159**:253–261.
3. Margulis AR, Burhenne HJ. *Practical Alimentary Tract Radiology.* Mosby Year Book, 1993.

8
Interventional radiology

Ken Mitchell

A. Biopsy
B. Drainage procedures
C. Vascular therapies
D. Speciality areas

There are a wide range of interventional procedures performed, and the number is constantly increasing. Because of the increasing complexity and rapidly advancing technology, many of the procedures are performed by speciality radiologists with expertise in the area involved. The availability of these interventional procedures is variable, but most radiologists will perform the basic procedures. The major procedures available are covered here.

A. BIOPSY

This is now a very common procedure. The usual sites include:

- lung
- abdominal
- mediastinal
- breast
- bone.

Two types of tissue sampling can be performed:

1. *Cytology* – aspiration of cells and fluid with fine-gauge needles.
2. *Histology* – actual tissue sampling with larger-bore needles, often with mechanical cutting needles.

Cytology is felt to be the safer procedure with smaller needles, but requires a good cytologist. Larger sample size is important in evaluating conditions such as lymphoma which require more advanced processing.

Indications:

- Diagnosis of a focal lesion.
- Primary or secondary malignancy, infection, or inflammation.

Patient preparation:

- May be inpatient or outpatient.
- Consent, coagulation profile.
- May also need sedation, iv access, antibiotics, and group-hold for high-risk procedures.
- Usually allowed fluids only for 4 hours before.

Method:

- Performed under imaging control with CT scanning, ultrasound, or fluoroscopy.
- Large variety of biopsy needles:
  (i) fine needle biopsy: 21–22 gauge;
  (ii) tissue core biopsy: 14–18 gauge.
- May use single needle, co-axial needle or mechanical assistant such as spring-loaded 'gun' device.
- After infiltration with local anaesthetic and antiseptic preparation, the needle tip is placed adjacent to or in the lesion. Fine-needle aspiration is applied with a 20 cc syringe and several advances into the lesion. A spring-loaded cutting needle will make a single pass into the lesion giving a 1–3 cm core of tissue.

Special problems:

- Lung biopsy: the lung may collapse due to pneumothorax on the initial puncture, so speed is essential in performing the biopsy.
- Bone biopsy: needles that cut through the bone are often necessary in lesions not causing marked bone destruction.

Post-procedure care:

- Patient is observed for 4–12 hours for bleeding.
- May be kept nil orally.
- Lung biopsy will require a chest X-ray to exclude pneumothorax.

Contra-indications:

- Bleeding disorders.
- Uncooperative patient.
- Inaccessible location – e.g. behind vascular structure, bowel, etc.

Complications:

- Bleeding.
- Sepsis.
- Leakage – bile, chyle, CFS, urine.

B. DRAINAGE PROCEDURES

This topic covers many different procedures. It includes abscesses, fluid collections, and decompression of biliary/renal tracts and stomach. It may be either a single 'in–out' aspiration or more complex placement of a special drainage catheter. The catheters can be placed percutaneously in the chest, liver, kidneys, and peritoneal cavity. Other avenues include transrectally, transvaginally, and transgastrically.

Indications:

Sepsis, poor surgical risk patient, pre-/post-operative problems, obstructed biliary or renal systems.

Method:

Imaging control:

- ultrasound
- CT
- fluoroscopy
- combination of above.
- (a) *Simple aspiration*: 22–18 gauge needle directed via 'safe' route under imaging control.
- (b) *Drainage catheter placement*: Either pushed in with a trochar or inserted over guiding wire initially placed through a needle. Often need to dilate tract with sequential dilators. From 6 French to 20 French size, catheters have various shapes and configurations to hold themselves in place. Most commonly they have a string which is pulled to form a loop.

Post-procedure care:

Close observation for sepsis and haemorrhage. Drainage catheters:

- free drainage
- low suction
- flush with saline and aspirate.
- Follow-up contrast study to assess result.
- Removal: cut string (if present) and pull catheters out when drainage finished.

Contra-indications:

Bleeding disorder.
Uncooperative patient.
No percutaneous access (very rare).

Complications:

Bleeding: false aneurysm may be treated by embolisation if fails to settle.
Sepsis: particularly in biliary or renal drainage, septic shock may be severe.
Failed drainage: catheter malposition needs adjustment or replacement.

C. VASCULAR THERAPIES

1. Angioplasty

Indications:

Relief of arterial ischaemia due to vascular narrowing – atherosclerosis, fibromuscular dysplasia, etc.
Most common site is the lower limb arteries, but is also applied to the aorta, renal, and mesenteric arteries and greater vessels of the arch of the aorta.

Patient preparation:

Requires hospitalisation and nil by mouth.
Coagulation profile and iv access; sedation; and group-holds. Aspirin is given as an antiplatelet agent.

Method:

Access is similar to arteriography (i.e. Seldinger technique). A percutaneous puncture of the femoral artery is made and a guide wire inserted – the angioplasty catheter can then be inserted over the wire (or through a sheath inserted over the wire).

The angioplasty catheter is like a standard angiographic catheter with a special balloon on it which is inflated via a side-port. The balloon has a specific size, length, and inflation pressure. The stenosis is 'crossed' with the guide wire and then by the balloon catheter which is inflated with diluted contrast media when in position. Several inflations lasting 15–60 seconds are performed, then a check angiogram to assess the results. An intravascular ultrasound catheter probe can also be used to assess the lumen.

Post-procedure care:

Nothing by mouth for 2 hours. Rest in bed for 12 hours. Close observation of the limb for delayed occlusion, observe groin for haematoma.

Contra-indications:

Bleeding disorder.
Multiple stenoses unsuitable.

Complications:

Arterial occlusion.
Thromboembolism.
Arterial dissection/rupture.
These may require urgent vascular surgery.
Recurrence of stenosis as a late complication.

2. Vascular stents

These are cylindrical metal mesh tubes which are used to keep the arterial lumen expanded. They are either self-expanding or need to be opened with a balloon catheter.

Indications:

For stenosis which is refractory to simple balloon angioplasty; complicated angioplasty (e.g. dissection); venous occlusive problems such as malignant SVC obstruction. The exact indications are still being investigated.

Patient preparation:

As for angioplasty.

Method:

Access as for angioplasty. The stent can be deployed either with the balloon dilatation or afterwards with a self-expanding stent.

Post-procedure care:

As for angioplasty.

Contra-indications:

As for angioplasty.

Complications:

As for angioplasty as well as stent dislodgement and embolisation.

3. Thrombolysis/atherectomy

Indications:

The role of thrombolysis is still being evaluated.

Recent improvements include the catheter used and the agents available. It may be indicated in acute thrombosis of arteries, grafts, and veins.

Patient preparation:

Nil by mouth, coagulation assessment, iv access.

Method:

The most recent advance is the combination of thrombolytic agents with mechanical dissolution of clots. A special catheter is placed in the clot and pulsed spray of a thrombolytic agent with advancement of the catheter is performed. This will expedite the process of thrombolysis. Agents used include streptokinase, urokinase and plasminogen activators (varying cost and efficiency).

Percutaneous atherectomy may be performed with mechanical cutting/drilling devices, laser devices, etc. Their role is still being investigated.

Post-procedure care:

Dosage of thrombolytic has to be monitored. Close observation of the patient for bleeding or re-thrombosis. Overnight infusions are sometimes used.
Monitoring in ICU is advised.

Contra-indications:

Recent surgery.
Peptic ulcer.
Intracranial lesions (risk of haemorrhage).
Allergy to agents.

Complications:

Haemorrhage – may be severe, especially cerebral.
Advantage of local infusion is reduced systemic effect.
Distal emboli.

4.   Vascular embolisation (*Fig. 8.1*)

Indications:

This covers a large number of procedures. It usually is transarterial, using a wide range of emboli materials.

Uses include: to stop bleeding, e.g. trauma, fistulas, arteriovenous malformations, aneurysms; to devascularise tumours; delivery of chemotherapeutic substances.

Patient preparation:

As for angioplasty.
Antibiotics and pain relief may be needed.
Risk of ischaemia needs to be discussed with patient.

Method:

The embolic material is delivered through a catheter: either a standard diagnostic angiographic catheter or specialised catheters, such as microcatheters, which can be coaxially placed through a larger guiding catheter and gain far more distal access. Embolic materials include: metal coils with or without thrombogenic fibres attached; particles (e.g. polyvinyl alcohol particles); glue (e.g. Superglue acrylates); detachable balloons – latex or silicon; gelfoam pledgets; IVC filters; chemotherapeutic agents; absolute alcohol; and many more substances. The type of material used depends on the site, flow characteristics, whether a permanent or temporary occlusion is required, and type of catheter in use. Personal preference is also important. The procedures usually require good imaging facilities, especially digital subtraction angiography, to monitor progress of embolisation and to diagnose complications.

Post-procedure care:

Rest in bed and close observation for problems of infarction and unwanted embolisation. Post-embolisation syndrome: pain and fever lasting several days.

Contra-indications:

Bleeding diathesis – relative.
Uncooperative patient.
Poor vascular access or unsatisfactory catheter placement.

Complications:

Infarction of non-pathological areas.
Infection of devascularised areas.

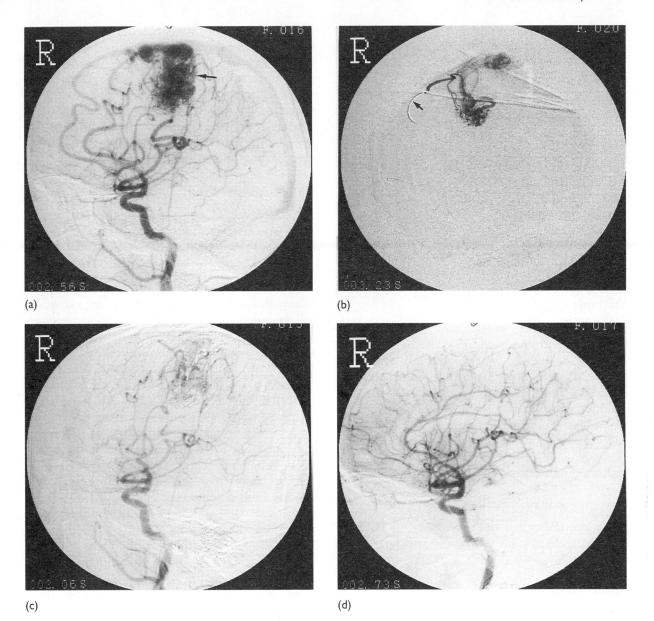

Fig. 8.1 Treatment of a cerebral AVM

a) Pre-embolisation

There is a large arteriovenous malformation (AVM) (arrow) supplied by branches of the right internal carotid artery.

b) Embolisation

A microcatheter (arrow) is seen in one of the arteries supplying the AVM. Cyanoacrylate glue is then injected, blocking off this artery.

c) Post-embolisation

The AVM shows decreased blood flow. Surgery may now be performed with much less risk of complication.

d) Post-surgery

The AVM has been successfully treated surgically.

Recanalised emboli: re-opened lesions.
Perforation of vessel: haemorrhage.

D. SPECIALITY AREAS

1. Neuroradiology

Indications:

Treatment or adjuvant treatment of vascular abnormalities and tumours.

Patient preparation:

Often under general anaesthetic.
Adequate informed consent mandatory.
Coagulation profile and iv access.

Method:

The rapid advances of technology have markedly advanced neurointerventions. The basic tool is the microcatheter which can be co-axially advanced from the groin deep into intracerebral arteries. The most common lesions treated include pre-operative embolisation of meningiomas and skull-base tumours with particles, balloon occlusions of carotico-cavernous fistulas, glue occlusion of intracerebral AVMs (*Fig. 8.1*) and coil embolisation of aneurysms.

Post-procedure care:

Often requires close observation in an ICU or high-dependency unit. Follow-up angiography to assess result.

Contra-indications:

Bleeding disorder.
Lack of vascular access, or unsuitable arterial anatomy.

Complications:

Stroke and death from inadvertent embolisation or rupture.

2. Hepatobiliary intervention

Indications:

Malignant biliary strictures/obstructions and, to a lesser degree, benign conditions can be managed either via ERCP or percutaneously, or a combination of the two.

Portal hypertension can also now be managed percutaneously with creation of a porto-caval shunt through the liver substance (TIPS – transjugular intrahepatic portosystemic shunt). This is really an extension of the transjugular liver biospy performed in patients for percutaneous biopsy due to bleeding disorders.

Patient preparation:

Nil orally, coagulation studies, iv access, antibiotics, adequate sedation.
Group-hold may be necessary.

Method:

Bilary drainage is performed as an extension of percutaneous transhepatic cholangiogram (PTC). The bile duct is punctured under fluoroscopy, a guide wire introduced, then a tract is dilated up over the wire. Finally, a drainage catheter (6–10 French) is placed. If felt to be indicated, and if the obstruction can be passed, a stent (similar to the vascular stents) can be placed opening up the obstruction and allowing removal of any external drains. This can give very good palliation. The TIPS procedure is performed via the jugular vein, punctured percutaneously with a long needle; cannulation of the portal vein through the liver from the hepatic vein means there cannot be any external bleeding in these sick patients with often advanced liver disease. The needle is replaced with a wire over which dilatation is performed. The portocaval shunt thus produced gives relief to either the variceal bleeding or intractable ascites. Percutaneous cholecystotomy can be performed in medically unfit patients with cholecystitis, especially acalculous type. Percutaneous calculus removal can also be performed.

Post-procedure care:

Close observation, often require ICU care.

Contra-indications:

Uncooperative patient.
Unsuitable anatomy.
Very poor risk patient.

Complications:

Sepsis, haemorrhage, biliary peritonitis.

---

3. Genito-urinary interventions

Indications:

Nephrostomy: obstructed collecting system, especially if septic or solitary kidney; failed retrograde stenting at cystoscopy; medically unfit patients.
Fallopian tube catheterisation: for infertility due to tubal obstruction.
Varicocele embolisation: for infertility from scrotal varicocele.

Patient preparation:

May need coagulation profile, iv access, antibiotics, and sedation.

Summary of method:

Nephrostomy: under fluoroscopy or ultrasound guidance; percutaneous needle placement, usually from postero-lateral approach, to the lower pole calyx; dilators and drainage catheter placed over guide wire. Further procedures such as stenting and stone removal can then be performed.
Fallopian tube catheterisation: a fine microcatheter is advanced under fluoroscopy through the uterine cavity into the tube; this breaks down any tubal obstructions with improved fertility.
Varicocele embolisation: percutaneous puncture, via the femoral vein; passage of a catheter into the IVC or left renal vein, and then retrogradely down the gonadal veins; occlusion is performed with coil or balloons. As the veins are incompetent without valves, the occlusion allows relief from the back pressure.

Post-procedure care:

Close observation.

Contra-indications:

Uncooperative patient.
Bleeding disorder.
Unsuitable anatomy.

Complications:

Sepsis, haemorrhage urinary leak.

9
Ultrasound

A. Physics and terminology
B. Further developments
C. Uses and advantages
D. Limitations and disadvantages

A. PHYSICS AND TERMINOLOGY

Ultrasound imaging uses ultra-high-frequency sound waves to produce cross-sectional images of the body. The basic component of the ultrasound probe is the piezoelectric crystal. Excitation of this crystal by electrical signals causes it to emit ultra-high-frequency sound waves: this is the *piezoelectric effect*. Sound waves are reflected back to the crystal by the various tissues of the body. These sound waves act on the piezoelectric crystal in the ultrasound probe to produce an electric signal, again by the piezoelectric effect. Analysis of this electric signal by a computer produces a cross-sectional image (*Fig. 9.1*).

Assorted body tissues produce various degrees of sound wave reflection and are said to be of different *echogenicity*. A tissue of high echogenicity reflects more sound than a tissue of low echnogenicity. The terms *hyperechoic* and *hypoechoic* are used to describe tissues of high and low

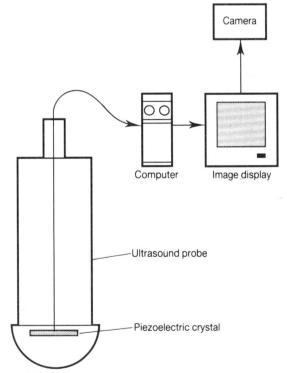

Fig. 9.1 Ultrasound
The piezo-electric crystal in the ultrasound probe is used to both transmit and receive the ultrasound waves. The returned signal is analysed by computer and displayed as an image.

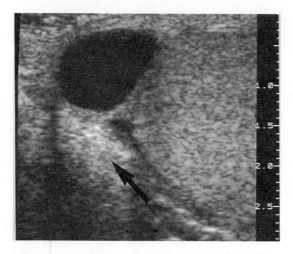

Fig. 9.2   Acoustic enhancement – epididymal cyst
Note: • well-defined hyperechoic area (arrow) deep to a
          simple cyst of the epididymis
        • normal testicle.

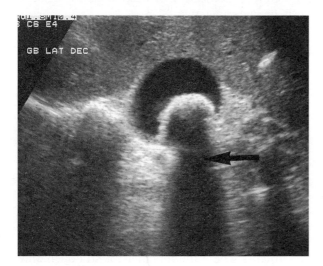

Fig. 9.3   Acoustic shadow – gallstone
Prominent acoustic shadow (arrow) deep to a large
gallstone.

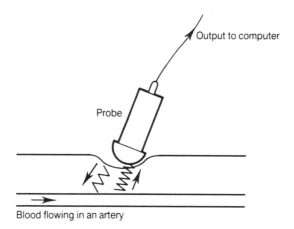

Fig. 9.4   Doppler ultrasound
In this diagram the blood flow is towards the ultrasound
probe. As such the returning signal is of higher frequency.
The frequency shift is analysed by computer and displayed
as a graph.

as black. Furthermore, because virtually all sound is transmitted through a fluid-containing area, tissues distal to such an area receive more sound and hence appear lighter. This effect is known as *acoustic enhancement* and is seen in tissues distal to the gallbladder, the urinary bladder, and simple cysts (*Fig. 9.2*). The reverse effect occurs with areas of sharply increased echogenicity where distal tissues receive little sound and are thus perceived as black. This phenomenon is known as *acoustic shadow* and is seen distal to gas containing areas, as well as gallstones, renal stones, and other areas of calcification (*Fig. 9.3*).

B. FURTHER DEVELOPMENTS

I. Doppler ultrasound

Anyone who has heard a police or ambulance siren speed past will be familiar with the *Doppler effect*, which describes the influence of a moving object on sound waves. An object travelling towards the listener causes sound waves to be compressed giving a higher frequency; an object travelling away from the listener gives a lower frequency.

The Doppler effect has been applied to ultrasound imaging. Flowing blood causes an alteration to the frequency of sound waves returning to the ultrasound probe. This frequency change or shift is calculated allowing quantitation of blood flow (*Fig. 9.4*).

echogenicity respectively. In producing an image hyperechoic tissues are shown as white or light grey, compared with hypoechoic tissues which are seen as dark grey. Examples of hyperechoic tissues include fat-containing masses and liver haemangiomata; lymphoma and fibroadenoma of the breast are examples of hypoechoic tissues.

Pure fluid reflects virtually no sound and is said to be *anechoic*. Fluid is seen on ultrasound images

Colour Doppler is an extension of these principles, in that blood flowing towards the transducer is coloured red; blood flowing away from the transducer is coloured blue. The colours are superimposed on the cross-sectional image allowing instant assessment of direction of flow. Colour Doppler is particularly useful in echocardiography and identifying very small vessels (e.g. calf veins, arcuate arteries in the kidneys).

2.   Intercavitary scanning

An assortment of probes are now available for imaging various body cavities and organs, most widely used and accepted being the use of transvaginal scanning. This technique allows more accurate assessment of gynaecological problems and of early pregnancy up to about 12 weeks' gestation. Transrectal probes are used to assess the prostate gland. Ultrasound crystals can be attached to endoscopes for assessment of tumours of the upper gastrointestinal tract. To date, this technique has found greatest application for staging of oesophageal tumours. Echocardiography can also be performed via an endoscopic probe sited in the oesophagus. This removes the problem of overlying ribs and lung which can obscure the heart when performing conventional echocardiography. Tiny ultrasound probes have also been developed for attachment to arterial catheters. These probes provide very accurate cross-sectional images of the arterial wall and, although expensive at present, are under continuing development.

3.   High frequency scanning

The use of high-frequency probes has opened up the area of musculo-skeletal ultrasound. This technique has found greatest application in the shoulder joint, specifically in the assessment of the rotator cuff. Most muscles and tendons of the body can also be examined for rupture, inflammation, tumour, etc. using ultrasound. Early work has been published on the use of ultra-high-frequency probes (20 mHz) in the use of skin conditions.

C. USES AND ADVANTAGES

The advantages of ultrasound are as follows:
1.   Lack of ionising radiation.
2.   Relative low cost.
3.   Portability of equipment.

Ultrasound scanning is applicable to the solid organs of the body. Initially, studies were directed to the liver, kidneys, spleen, and pancreas and to the pelvic organs. Higher-frequency, smaller probes led to the use of ultrasound in diseases of the thryoid, breast, and testes, as well as the musculo-skeletal system as above. The lack of ionising radiation is a particular advantage in the assessment of pregnancy and in paediatrics. Used in conjunction with Doppler, ultrasound is now used in a wide variety of cardiovascular applications including: echocardiography; assessment of carotid, renal, mesenteric, and peripheral arteries for stenosis; assessment of deep veins for thrombosis or incompetence.

D. LIMITATIONS AND DISADVANTAGES

Ultrasound cannot penetrate gas or bone. Hence lesions lying behind or within gas or bone cannot be visualised. Therefore ultrasound is not used for pulmonary conditions and bowel gas may obscure structures deep in the abdomen (e.g. the pancreas or renal arteries). Bone lesions are not usually amenable to assessment with ultrasound. Similarly, the intracranial contents cannot be examined due to the overlying skull vault. The two exceptions to this are:
1.   Infants where the fontanelle is still open and provides a 'window'.
2.   Intraoperative localisation of brain lesions during craniotomy.

Further Reading

1.   Foley WD, Erickson SJ. Color Doppler flow imaging. AJR 1991;**156**:3–13.
2.   Nyberg DA, Hill LM, Bohm-Velez M, Mendelson EB. *Transvaginal Ultrasound*. Mosby Year Book, 1992.
3.   Van Holsbeeck M, Introcaso JH. *Musculoskeletal Ultrasound*. Mosby Year Book, 1991.
4.   Wells PNT. Doppler ultrasound in medical diagnosis. *British Journal of Radiology* 1989;**62**:399–420.
5.   Zwiebel WJ (ed.). *Introduction to Vascular Ultrasonography*, 2nd edn. Grune and Stratton, 1986.

10
Computed tomography (CT)

A. Physics and terminology
B. Further developments
C. Uses and advantages
D. Limitations and disadvantages

A. PHYSICS AND TERMINOLOGY

Computed tomography (CT) is an imaging technique whereby cross-sectional images are obtained with the use of X-rays. The patient passes through a gantry which rotates around at the level of interest. The gantry has an X-ray tube on one side and a set of detectors on the other. Information from the detectors is analysed by computer and displayed as an image. Owing to the use of computer analysis, a much greater array of densities can be displayed than on conventional X-ray films. This allows differentiation of solid organs from each other and from pathological processes such as tumour or fluid collections. It also makes CT extremely sensitive to the presence of minute amounts of calcium or contrast material (*Fig. 10.1*).

As with plain radiography, high-density objects cause more attenuation of the X-ray beam and are therefore displayed as lighter grey than objects of lower density. White and light grey objects are therefore said to be of 'high attenuation'; dark grey and black objects are said to be of 'low attenuation'. Furthermore, the image information can be manipulated by the computer to display the various tissues of the body. This is called 'altering the window settings'. For example, in chest CT where a wide range of tissue densities is present, a good image of the mediastinal structures shows no lung details. By setting a lung window the lung parenchyma is seen in remarkable detail, though the mediastinal structures are poorly differentiated (*Fig. 10.2*). This technique can also be used to accentuate a subtle difference in tissue density. For example, the use of 'liver windows' allows greater differentiation of tumours whose tissue density closely approximates that of surrounding normal liver tissue.

Intravenous contrast is used in CT for a number of reasons, as follows:

1. Differentiation of normal blood vessels from abnormal masses (e.g. hilar vessels versus lymph nodes).
2. To make an abnormality more apparent (e.g. liver metastases).
3. To demonstrate the vascular nature of a mass and thus aid in characterisation (*Fig. 10.3*).

81

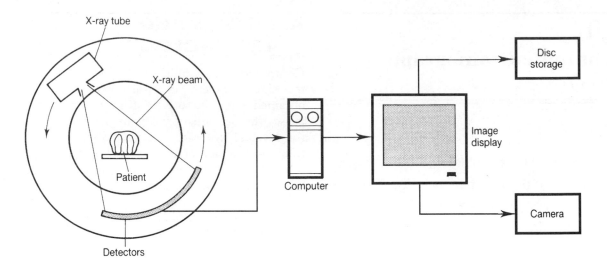

Fig. 10.1   Computed tomography – CT.

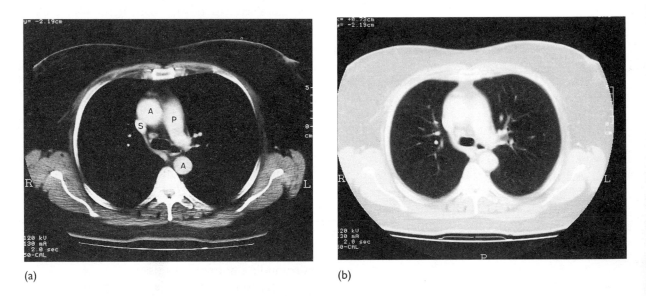

(a)   (b)

Fig. 10.2   CT windows

a) Mediastinal window

Note that mediastinal anatomy is well shown; no lung detail can be seen.

Note also the following structures:

- aorta: (A)
- SVC: (S)
- pulmonary artery: (P).

b) Lung window

Note that the vascular anatomy of the lungs is now well seen.

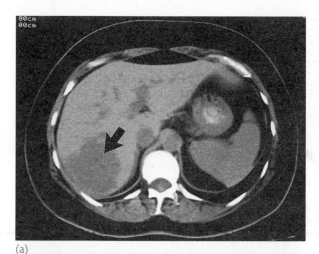

(a)

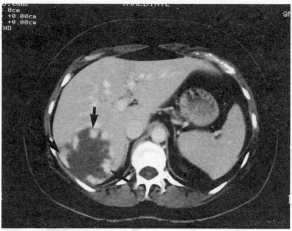

(b)

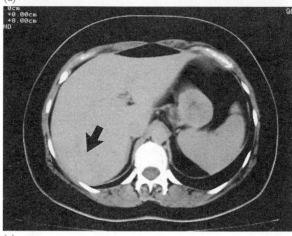

(c)

Fig. 10.3   Contrast CT – liver haemangioma
a) Pre-contrast scan
Note: • large mass in the right lobe of the liver (arrow)
         • low attenuation compared with surrounding normal liver.
b) Immediate post-contrast scan
Note: • contrast in aorta, IVC, and portal vein branches
         • dense contrast enhancement of the periphery of the mass (arrows).
c) 50-minute post-contrast scan
The mass is now uniformly enhanced (arrow), so its density is equal to that of normal liver tissue. This is a typical enhancement pattern for haemangioma of the liver.

Oral contrast is also used for abdomen CT to allow differentiation of normal enhancing bowel loops from abnormal masses or fluid collections. For detailed examination of the pelvis, rectal contrast and a vaginal tampon will aid in the differentiation of these structures from pathology.

B. FURTHER DEVELOPMENTS

Helical (spiral) CT

CT scanners have now been developed which allow continuous acquisition of data as the patient passes through the gantry. These machines differ from conventional scanners in that the tube and detectors rotate without stops as the patient passes through on the scanning table. In this way, a volumetric set of data is obtained which has a spiral configuration (*Fig. 10.4*). This

remarkable advance has been due to a number of factors:

1. Better X-ray tube technology.
2. Better detector technology.
3. More sophisticated computer software allowing calculation of the complex data.
4. Development of slip-ring technology. The X-ray tube and detectors rotate on a number of slip-rings; these are metal rings which have three functions:
   (i) supply of high-voltage electricity to the X-ray tube;
   (ii) supply of low-voltage electricity for various control mechanisms;
   (iii) transfer of digital data from the detectors to the computer.

The major advantages of helical scanning over conventional scanning are:

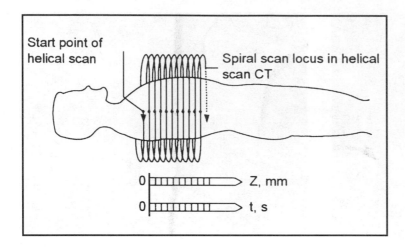

Fig. 10.4 Spiral CT
A schematic diagram to show the scanning method of spiral CT. 'Z' represents the Z-plane, i.e. the direction of passage of the patient through the scanner; 't, s' equals time in seconds. Obviously the scanner spins in a circle. The spiral 'shape' of acquired data is due to movement of the patient through the spinning gantry. (Courtesy GE Medical Systems Australia Pty Ltd)

1. Increased speed of examination.
2. Rapid examination at optimal levels of intravenous contrast concentration.
3. Images can be retrospectively reconstructed at any desired level.
4. The continuous nature of data allows accurate high-quality 3D reconstruction. This has many applications, both potential and currently realised e.g. planning of cranial, facial reconstruction surgery; repair of fractures in complex areas e.g.acetabulum; CT angiography i.e. display of blood vessels such as the aorta prior to surgery.

C. USES AND ADVANTAGES

The first CT scanners developed, due to their small size, were used only for examination of the head and its contents. With the development of larger scanners, CT is now applied to all areas of the body. CT is the modality of choice for the mediastinum and for many pulmonary conditions. It is also the method of choice for examination of the retroperitoneum and for many disorders of the solid abdominal and pelvic organs. It is excellent in the delineation of bony pathology and it has been used extensively for spinal diseases despite some limitations, as outlined below.

D. LIMITATIONS AND DISADVANTAGES

Disadvantages of CT relate to its use of ionising radiation, hazards of intravenous contrast, lack of portability of equipment, and its relatively high cost.

A number of areas of the body are imaged relatively poorly with CT. These include the pituitary fossa and the posterior intracranial fossa where artefact from adjacent bony structures obscures normal anatomy. MRI is the modality of choice for these areas. In the spine, despite its excellent soft tissue contrast capabilities, CT is unable to differentiate spine/spinal cord/nerve roots from surrounding CSF (unless the CSF has been opacified by myelography which is obviously invasive). For this reason, MRI is the imaging modality of choice in the spine.

Internal gastrointestinal pathology, like polyps, ulcero-inflammatory diseases, and tumours, are not usually seen by CT unless there is associated bowel wall thickening or pericolonic masses or fluid collections. CT imaging is usually limited to the transverse (axial plane).

Exceptions relate to areas of the body that can be tilted in the gantry (e.g. the head or ankles) to give coronal scans. Helical scanning allows reconstructive imaging in the sagittal plane (e.g. for assessment of the spine), though the images are of relatively poor quality compared with MRI.

Further Reading

1. Lee JKT, Sagel SS, Stanley RJ. *Computed Body Tomography with MRI Correlation*, 2nd edn. Raven Press, 1989.
2. Lee SH, Rao KCVG, Zimmerman RA. *Cranial MRI and CT*, 3rd edn. McGraw-Hill, 1992.
3. Zeman RK, Fox SH, Silverman PM *et al.* Helical (spiral) CT of the Abdomen. *AJR* 1993;**160**:719–725.

11

Scintigraphy – nuclear medicine

A. Physics and terminology
B. Uses and advantages
C. Limitations and disadvantages
D. Further developments

A. PHYSICS AND TERMINOLOGY

Scintigraphy refers to the use of gamma radiation to form images following the injection of various radio-pharmaceuticals. The keyword to understanding scintigraphy is 'radio-pharmaceutical', where 'radio' part refers to the emitter of gamma rays (i.e. a radionuclide). The most commonly used radionuclide in clinical practice is technetium, written in this text as ^{99m}Tc., where 99 is the atomic mass; and the small 'm' stands for 'metastable', the property which causes the material to emit gamma radiation. Metastable means that the technetium atom has two basic energy states: high and low. As the technetium passes from the high-energy state to the low-energy state, it emits a packet of energy in the form of a gamma ray which has an energy of 140 keV (kiloelectron volts) (*Fig. 11.1*). The gamma rays are detected by a gamma camera which converts the absorbed energy of the radiation to

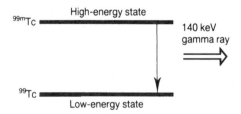

Fig. 11.1 Gamma ray production
The metastable atom ^{99m}Tc in passing from the high energy state to the lower energy state releases gamma radiation which has a peak energy of 140 K.e.V. This makes it very suitable for use in imaging. ^{99m}Tc has a half life of about 6 hours.

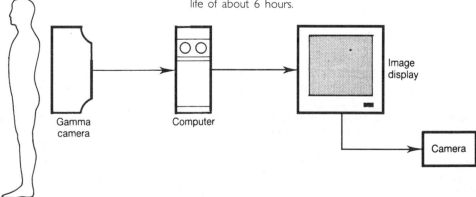

Fig. 11.2 Scintigraphy.

an electric signal. This signal is analysed by a computer and displayed as an image (*Fig. 11.2*). Other commonly used radionuclides include gallium citrate (^{67}Ga), thallium (^{201}Tl), indium (^{111}In), and iodine (^{131}I).

'Pharmaceutical' refers to the compound to which the radionuclide is bound. This compound will depend on the area to be examined. For example, sulphur colloid is taken up by the reticulo-endothelial cells of the liver and spleen and is therefore used in imaging these organs. For some applications a pharmaceutical is not required. An example would be the use of free technetium (^{99m}Tc), referred to as pertechnetate, for thyroid scanning. A list of the common radio-pharmaceuticals and their applications is provided in Table 11.1.

Areas of high uptake of pharmaceutical and therefore of the radionuclide to which it is bound show resultant high emission of gamma rays.

These areas are referred to as 'hot'. Areas of low uptake are referred to as photon-deficient or 'cold'.

B. USES AND ADVANTAGES

The main advantages of scintigraphy are:

1. Highly sensitive, e.g. early osteomyelitis may not be visible on plain films for 7–10 days while scintigraphy will be positive at the time of presentation.
2. Functional information is provided as well as anatomical information, e.g. DTPA renal scans provide information on renal function, as well as renal size and drainage of the collecting systems.

The common radio-pharmaceuticals and their applications are summarised below:

Organ	Radio-pharmaceutical	Clinical application
Kidneys	^{99m}Tc-DTPA	Renal function, anatomy, drainage of collecting systems
	^{99m}Tc-DMSA	Cortical scars in children with urinary tract infection
	^{99m}Tc in saline passed into the bladder by catheter	Vesico-ureteric reflux in children with urinary tract infection
Bone	^{99m}Tc-MDP	Bone metastases, activity of bone lesions, stress fractures
Lungs	Ventilation: ^{99m}Tc-DTPA aerosol Perfusion: ^{99m}Tc-MAA	Pulmonary embolism
Liver/spleen	^{99m}Tc-colloid	Liver/spleen masses
Bile ducts	^{99m}Tc-HIDA	Acute cholecystitis, biliary obstruction, biliary atresia, post-liver transplant
Thyroid	^{99m}Tc	Thyroid function, thyroiditis, function of thyroid masses, location of aberrant thyroid tissue
Gated cardiac study	Stannous pyro-phosphate to reduce Hb then ^{99m}Tc which binds reduced Hb and thus red blood cells	Left ventricular ejection fraction, localised wall motion defects (e.g post-infarct)
Bleeding studies	^{99m}Tc labelled red blood cells as for gated cardiac study	Acute gastrointestinal bleeding
Myocardium	^{201}Tl	Ischaemic/infarcted myocardium
Parathyroid	^{99m}Tc and ^{201}Tl	Hyperparathyroidism
Adrenal medulla	^{131}I-MIBG	Localisation of phaeochromocytoma
CSF	^{111}In-DTPA	Differentiation of communicating hydrocephalus from cerebral atrophy

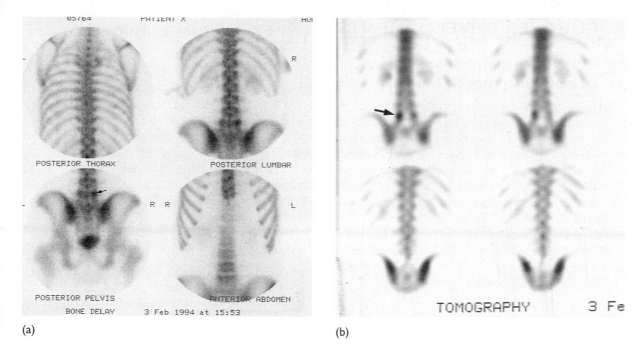

(a)

(b)

Fig. 11.3 SPECT scan – pars interarticularis defect
a) Conventional bone scan
There is a subtle area of increased uptake of radiopharmaceutical in the region of the right pars interarticularis of L5 (arrow).
b) SPECT scan
SPECT scans in the coronal plane give a much better demonstration of the 'hot spot' in L5 indicating a pars interarticularis defect (arrow).

Gallium (^{67}Ga) scanning is used in a number of clinical situations. Gallium is bound to plasma proteins, most strongly to transferin. It is also taken up by white blood cells. Scanning is performed at 24, 48, and occasionally 72 hours post-injection. The three most common indications for gallium scanning are:

1. To localise occult infection usually in a patient with pyrexia of unknown origin or suspected abdominal abscess not localised by CT or ultrasound.
2. To confirm or deny that an abnormality seen on other studies (e.g. plain films or ^{99m}Tc-MDP bone scan) is infective in nature.
3. In staging and follow-up of Hodgkin's disease, although this role is usually performed by CT.

C. LIMITATIONS AND DISADVANTAGES

The main disadvantage of scintigraphy is its non-specificity. To take a common example, an isolated 'hot spot' on a bone scan could be due to infection, trauma, or neoplasia and correlation with clinical history and other imaging studies is of paramount importance. On the other hand, multiple 'hot spots' on the bone scan of an elderly man being staged for prostatic carcinoma are easily diagnosed as skeletal metastases. Furthermore, given the high sensitivity of bone scans, a normal study in such a patient virtually excludes skeletal metastatic disease.

Other disadvantages relate to the use of ionising radiation, the cost of equipment, and the extra care required in handling radioactive materials.

D. FURTHER DEVELOPMENTS

I. SPECT (single photon emission computed tomography)

This is a technique whereby the computer is programmed to analyse data coming from a single depth within the patient. In this way, cross-sectional scans analogous to plain tomography are obtained. This technique allows greater sensitivity in the detection of subtle lesions overlain by other active structures (e.g. pars interarticularis defects in the lower spine). The main applications of SPECT are in bone scanning, ^{201}Tl cardiac scanning, and in cerebral perfusion studies (*Fig. 11.3*).

2. PET (positron emission tomography)

This technique uses positron-emitting radionuclides. Research indicates that PET can produce good functional information and may have uses particularly in the brain for assessment of epilepsy, degenerative cerebral conditions, and in various psychiatric conditions. Unfortunately, the radionuclides used for PET are very short-lived and must be produced by a cyclotron. As such, PET is yet to find wide acceptance beyond research institutions.

Further Reading

1. Datz FL. *Handbooks in Radiology: Nuclear Medicine.* Mosby Year Book, 1988.
2. Ott RJ. Nuclear medicine in the 1990s: a quantitative physiological approach. *British Journal of Radiology* 1989;**62**:421–432.

12
Magnetic resonance imaging (MRI)

A. Physics and terminology
B. Uses and advantages
C. Limits and disadvantages
D. Further developments

A. PHYSICS AND TERMINOLOGY

MRI has over the past ten years become accepted as a powerful imaging tool. It uses the magnetic properties of the hydrogen atom to produce images. The physics of MRI is extremely complex and a full discussion would require a much larger book than this (and another author!). The following is a brief summary of the physical principles behind MRI.

The nucleus of the hydrogen atom is a single proton. Being a spinning, charged particle, it has magnetic properties and, for the sake of discussion, may be thought of as a small bar magnet with North and South poles (*Fig. 12.1*). The first step in MRI is the application of a strong, external magnetic field. For this purpose, the patient is placed within a large magnet, either a permanent or superconductive magnet.

The hydrogen atoms within the patient align in a direction either parallel or anti-parallel to the strong external field. A greater proportion align in the parallel direction, so that the net vector of their alignment, and therefore the net magnetic vector, will be in the direction of the external field (*Fig. 12.2*).

Though aligned in a strong magnetic field, the hydrogen nuclei do not lie motionless. Each nucleus spins around the line of the field in a

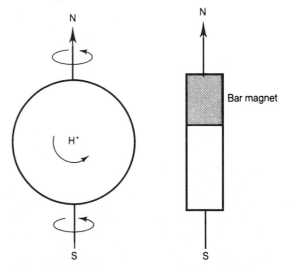

Fig. 12.1 The spinning hydrogen atom
The hydrogen atom being a spinning charged particle, has a small magnetic field, analagous to a bar magnet.

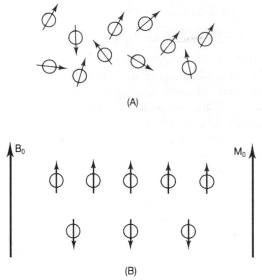

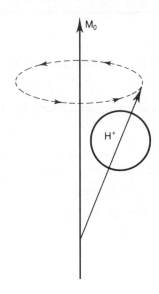

Fig. 12.2　Effect of application of a strong external magnetic field.

In a), the hydrogen atoms are randomly aligned in the normal resting state. In b), a strong external magnetic field, Bo, is applied. The atoms align either parallel or anti-parallel to this field. The majority align parallel so their net magnetic vector, M_0, is in the same direction as the external field, B_0.

Fig. 12.3　Precession
The hydrogen atom spins around the line of the magnetic field in a motion called precession at a frequency call the Larmor frequency.

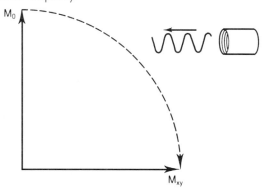

Fig. 12.4　Application of the RF pulse
Application of a pulsed magnetic field at 90° to the original field and at the Larmor frequency causes the net magnetic vector of the hydrogen atoms, M_0, to rotate through 90° onto the xy plane.

motion known as *precession* (*Fig. 12.3*). The frequency of precession is an inherent property of the hydrogen atom in a given magnetic field and is known as the *Larmor frequency*. The Larmor frequency therefore changes in proportion to magnetic field strength. It is of the order of 10^7 per second, i.e. 10 MHz (megaherz), a frequency in the same part of the electromagnetic spectrum as radio-waves.

A second magnetic field is now applied at right-angles to the original external field. This second magnetic field is applied at the same frequency as the Larmor frequency and is known as the *radiofrequency pulse* (RF pulse). The RF pulse is applied by a second magnetic coil – the RF coil. The RF pulse causes the net magnetisation vector of the hydrogen atoms to turn towards the transverse plane, i.e. a plane at right-angles to the direction of the original, strong external field (*Fig. 12.4*). As such, the RF pulse adds energy to the system. Following cessation of the RF pulse, the extra energy is dissipated to the surrounding chemical lattice in a process known as *T1 relaxation*. In addition, the RF pulse brings the precessing protons into phase, i.e. their spins

are now in synchrony. The process of dephasing, which occurs due to tiny inhomogeneities in the nuclear magnetic environment, is known as *T2 relaxation*.

The component of the net magnetisation vector in the transverse plane induces a current in magnetic coils known as *radiofrequency*, or *RF receiver coils*. This current is known as the *MR signal* and is the basis for formation of an image. Note that the MR signal can be produced only when the precession of the spinning protons is in phase. Complex computer analysis of the MR

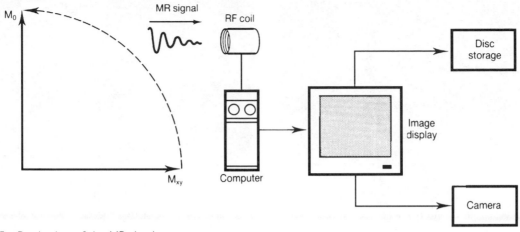

Fig. 12.5 Production of the MR signal
When the RF pulse is switched off, the net magnetisation vector returns to its original direction and emits a signal which is received by the RF coil. This signal is analysed by computer to produce an image.

signal from the RF receiver coils is used to produce an *MR image (Fig. 12.5)*.

Whereas CT depends on tissue density and ultrasound on tissue echogenicity, much of the complexity of MRI arises from the fact that the MR signal depends on many varied properties of substances being examined. These properties include:

- Proton density.
- The chemical environment of the hydrogen atoms (e.g. whether in free water or bound by fat).
- Flow (e.g. in blood or CSF).
- Magnetic susceptibility.
- T1 relaxation time.
- T2 relaxation time.

By altering the duration and amplitude of the RF pulse, as well as the timing and repetition of its application, various sequences have been developed to use and accentuate these various properties. The most common types of images produced have been:

(a) *T1 weighted*: excellent anatomical definition, though with lower sensitivity to pathology.
(b) *T2 weighted*: highly sensitive to the presence of pathology.

Numerous other image types are now used. A common example is fat suppression sequences which are excellent for demonstrating pathology in areas containing a lot of fat (e.g. the orbits and bone marrow). Note that in viewing MRI images white or light grey areas are referred to as 'high signal'; dark grey or black areas are referred to as 'low signal'. On certain sequences flowing blood is seen as a black area referred to as a 'flow void'.

B. USES AND ADVANTAGES

The main advantages of MRI are as follows.

1. Excellent soft tissue contrast

- As explained above, MRI uses many varied properties of matter in the generation of an image.

2. Lack of artefact due to adjacent bones

- This makes MRI the imaging modality of choice in areas such as the posterior fossa and pituitary fossa where the quality of CT images is degraded by artefact (*Fig. 12.6*).

3. Multiplanar capabilities

- MRI is able to obtain images in any plane. The sagittal plane is particularly useful for the spine and this property, combined with the excellent soft tissue

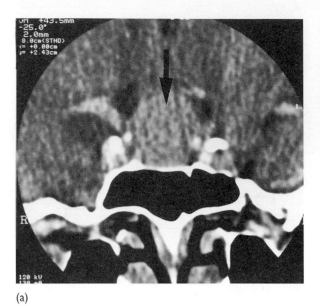

(a)

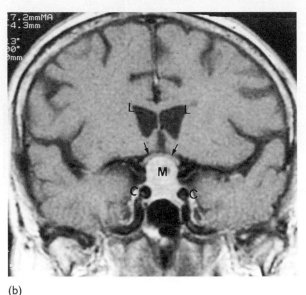

(b)

Fig. 12.6 Pituitary adenoma
a) CT
CT in the coronal plane demonstrates a mass arising from
the pituitary fossa (arrow).

b) MRI T1-weighted image with contrast
Anatomical detail is much better than with CT.
Note: • mass arising from the pituitary fossa (M)
       • compressed optic chiasm (arrows)
       • carotid arteries on either side (C)
       • lateral ventricles (L).

contrast, makes MRI the modality of choice for imaging of spinal disorders. Multiple planes are also useful in the musculo-skeletal system, e.g. sagittal and coronal planes for the knee, coronal and oblique planes for the shoulder.

4. Lack of ionising radiation

In summary, MRI is the imaging modality of choice for most brain and spine disorders. It has also found wide acceptance in the assessment of musculo-skeletal disorders. Although excellent for visualisation of the heart, echo-cardiography is more widely used as it produces functional as well as anatomical information. MRI has not displaced other modalities, such as CT, ultra-sound, and endoscopy, in the imaging of most thoracic and abdominal disorders.

C. LIMITATIONS AND DISADVANTAGES

1. Cost

- The equipment for MRI is very expensive. Running and maintenance costs are also high. Potential benefits to patient these costs.

2. Artefacts

- Although free of artefacts from bony structures, a wide variety of artefacts do occur in MRI.

3. Metal foreign objects

- MRI is potentially hazardous for patients with metal foreign bodies in the eyes and for patients with ferromagnetic intracranial aneurysm clips. MRI is contraindicated in patients with cardiac pacemakers and cochlear implants. Also artefacts from even small fragments of metal from orthopaedic surgery cause serious image degradation, though this is minimised with the use of titanium.

4. Reduced sensitivity for certain substances

- MRI is less sensitive than CT in the detection of small amounts of calcification and in the detection of acute haemorrhage. As such, CT is still the imaging modality of choice for the assessment of acute subarachnoid haemorrhage and for acute head injury.

5. Fine bone detail

- MRI is unable to provide the degree of bone detail possible with CT, although it is more sensitive in the detection of infiltrative disorders of bone marrow.

D. FURTHER DEVELOPMENTS

1. Contrast material

Although not as widely used as in CT imaging, intravenous contrast is now available for MRI. Gadolinium (Gd) is a paramagnetic substance which causes increased signal on T1-weighted images. Unbound Gadolinium is highly toxic. For this reason, binding agents are required for in vivo use. The most common of these is diethyltri-aminepentaacetic acid (DTPA): Gd-DTPA is non-toxic and used in a dose of 0.1 mmol per kilogram.

The main indications for the use of Gd-DTPA are as follows:
(a) *Brain (Fig. 12.7)*
- Multiple lesions (e.g. metastases, multiple sclerosis).
- Selected tumours (e.g. acoustic neuroma, meningioma).
- Tumour residuum/recurrence following treatment.
(b) *Spine*
- Metastases: intraspinal, CSF.
- Tumour recurrence.
- Post-operative to differentiate fibrosis from recurrent disc protrusion.
- Infection.
- Selected tumours (e.g. neurofibroma).
(c) *Musculoskeletal system*
- Soft tissue tumours.
- Intra-articular Gd-DTPA in subtle shoulder disorders.

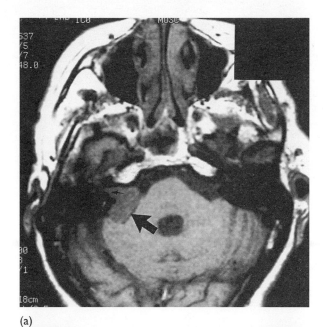

(a)

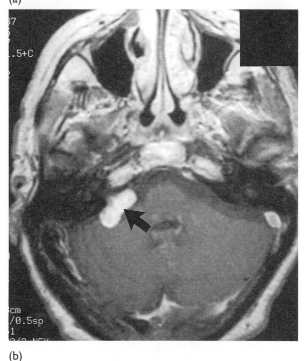

(b)

Fig. 12.7 MRI with contrast – acoustic neuroma
a) T1-weighted scan, axial plane
Right cerebello-pontine angle mass (large arrow). The mass shows lateral extension into the internal auditory meatus (small arrow), typical of acoustic neuroma.
b) T1-weighted scan with contrast, axial plane
The cerebello-pontine angle mass shows quite marked enhancement (arrow).

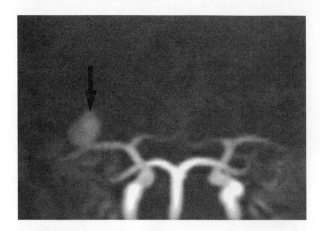

Fig. 12.8   MRA – berry aneurysm
Magnetic resonance angiography of the intracranial circulation shows an aneurysm of the right middle cerebral artery (arrow).

2.   Magnetic resonance angiography (MRA)

With varying sequences, flowing blood can be shown as either signal void (i.e. black), or increased signal (i.e. white). Computer recon-

struction techniques allow the display of blood vessels in 3D, and allow viewing of the blood vessels from any angle. Indications would include: imaging of the carotid arteries for stroke, TIA, aneurysm, AVM, etc.; imaging of the peripheral vessels for claudication. Many workers feel that MRA will largely replace diagnostic angiography in the not too distant future (*Fig. 12.8*).

3.   Fast imaging

New, complex sequences are under constant development. Much research is currently directed at very rapid image acquisition.

Further Reading

1. Higgins CB, Hricak H, Helms CA. *Magnetic Resonance Imaging of the Body*, 2nd edn. Raven Press, 1992.
2. Lee SH, Rao KCVG, Zimmerman RA. *Cranial MRI and CT*, 3rd edn. McGraw-Hill, 1992.
3. Siani S, Modic MT, Hamm B, Hahn PF. Advances in contrast-enhanced MR imaging. *AJR* 1991; **156**: 235–254.
4. Villafana T. Fundamental physics of magnetic resonance imaging. *Radiological Clinics of North America* 1988;**26**:701–715.

SECTION IV

Imaging in clinical practice

13

Cardiovascular system

A. Ischaemic heart disease/myocardial infarct
B. Congenital heart disease
C. Deep venous thrombosis (DVT)
D. Pulmonary embolism
E. Abdominal aortic aneurysm
F. Aortic dissection
G. Peripheral arterial disease
H. Hypertension

A. ISCHAEMIC HEART DISEASE/MYOCARDIAL INFARCT

1. Chest X-ray

- Normal in uncomplicated cases.
- Signs of cardiac failure (i.e. cardiac enlargement, pulmonary oedema, pleural effusions).
- Rarely signs of left ventricular aneurysm may be seen (i.e. abnormal bulging contour of the left heart border associated with calcification).

2. Coronary angiography (*Fig. 13.1*)

- To date, coronary angiography is the only imaging method available to accurately delineate the coronary arteries.
- Combined with intervention (i.e. angioplasty or streptokinase infusion).

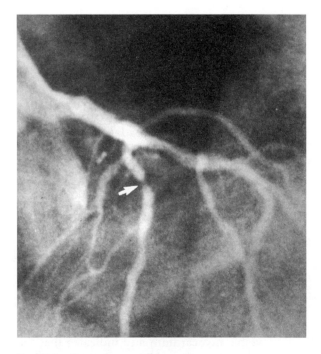

Fig. 13.1   Coronary artery stenosis
Left coronary angiogram shows a localised stenosis of the anterior descending branch (arrow).

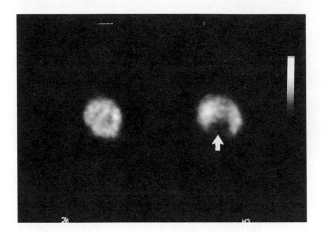

Fig. 13.2 Cardiac ischaemia – thallium scan
At rest (left) there is a normal distribution of thallium.
The exercise scan (right) shows a large defect at the
cardiac apex indicating an area of ischaemia (arrow).

3. Scintigraphy

(a) Thallium (^{201}Tl) exercise test (*Fig. 13.2*):

- Used to differentiate viable from non-viable myocardium and hence identify those patients who would benefit from coronary revascularisation procedures such as angioplasty or bypass graft.
- Following injection with ^{201}Tl, imaging is performed immediately after exercise and then repeated 4 hours later.
- Areas of infarct show as defects (i.e. 'cold' spots on both series).
- Areas of ischaemia show as defects on the post-exercise series which later fill in on the delayed series.
- The procedure has been modified recently, with a second dose of ^{201}Tl being administered under resting conditions; this results in a significant uptake in 50% of so-called 'fixed defects' on the 4 hour delayed scan; this modification therefore provides more accurate delineation of viable myocardium and indicates that the extent of non-viable myocardium had been overestimated by the initial Thallium technique.

(b) Infarct imaging;

- ^{99m}Tc labelled phosphates.
- Infarct shows as an area of increased uptake (i.e. a 'hot' spot).

(c) Gated cardiac scan:

- ^{99m}Tc labelled red blood cells.
- Left ventricular ejection fraction (i.e. measurement of left ventricular function).
- Regional wall motion analysis.
- Left ventricular aneurysm.

4. Echocardiography

- Good assessment of left ventricular ejection fraction.
- Complications (e.g. papillary muscle rupture, ventricular septal defect, left ventricular aneurysm, pericardial effusion).

B. CONGENITAL HEART DISEASE

I. Plain films

Plain-film assessment of suspected congenital heart disease is extremely difficult as the changes are often non-specific. In addition, plain films are often normal or exhibit only subtle changes, despite the presence of a complex cardiac defect. The following approach would be recommended in the assessment of chest X-ray for suspected congenital heart disease:

- Cardiac size.
- Specific chamber enlargement (see chest X-ray, chapter 4).
- Cardiac situs.
- Situs of other structures (i.e. aortic arch, stomach).
- Pulmonary vascular patterns.
  - (i) plethora (i.e. increased pulmonary blood flow as occurs in left to right shunts such as ASD, VSD, and PDA): dilated and tortuous pulmonary arteries; increased number of pulmonary arteries (*Fig. 13.3*).

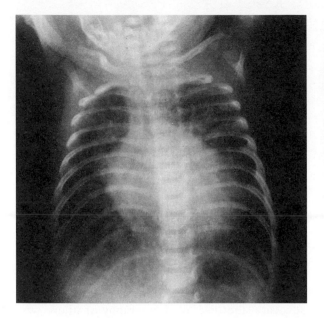

Fig. 13.3   Pulmonary plethora – transposition of the great vessels
Note: • increased number and size of pulmonary arteries
• cardiomegaly with an egg shaped heart
• narrow superior mediastinum due to overlap of the transposed aorta and pulmonary artery, plus a degree of thymic hypoplasia.

Pulmonary plethora may be due to left to right shunt as occurs with ASD, VSD, and PDA. It may also be associated with cyanotic conditions such as transposition of the great vessels or total anomalous pulmonary venous drainage.

      (ii) oligaemia (i.e. decreased pulmonary blood flow as occurs in pulmonary hypertension and in right outflow tract obstruction: Fallot's tetralogy, Ebstien's anomaly, pulmonary atresia, tricuspid atresia) (*Fig. 13.4*).
• Cardiac failure (i.e. pulmonary oedema, pleural effusions).
• Skeletal changes:
    (i) scoliosis;
    (ii) rib notching as occurs in aortic coarctation.

2.   Echocardiography

• Has replaced angiocardiography.
• Non-invasive assessment of:
    (i) cardiac anatomy;

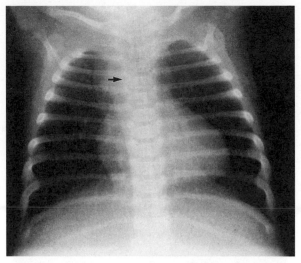

Fig. 13.4   Pulmonary oligaemia – Fallot's tetralogy
Note: • thin pulmonary vessels indicating decreased pulmonary blood flow
• apex of heart displaced upwards and laterally indicating right ventricular hypertrophy
• right-sided aortic arch as occurs in 30% of patients with Fallot's tetralogy (arrow).

    (ii) valvular function;
    (iii) shunts (e.g. VSD, ASD);
    (iv) anatomy of aortic root, aortic arch, and main pulmonary arteries.

3.   MRI

• Good anatomical information.
• May supplement echocardiography in complex cases.

C.   DEEP VENOUS THROMBOSIS (DVT)

1.   Ultrasound

• Non-invasive, painless, and inexpensive.
• Reliable for femoral and popliteal veins.
• Use of colour Doppler allows reasonably accurate delineation of calf veins.
• May detect conditions producing clinical signs and symptoms similar to DVT (e.g. ruptured Baker's cyst).
• Signs of DVT:
    (i) non-compressibility of veins;

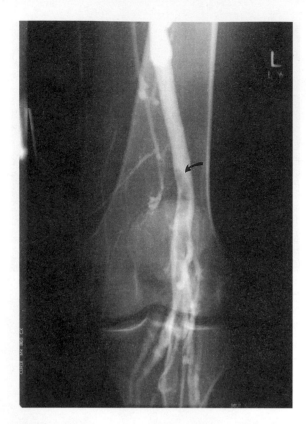

Fig. 13.5 Deep venous thrombosis (DVT) – venogram
DVT is seen as a filling defect in the popliteal veins
(arrow).
Note normal filling of more proximal deep veins.

Many clinicians do not consider thrombus limited to the calf veins important as it is felt that significant pulmonary embolism from these small vessels is rare. Adherents to this philosophy would not anticoagulate a patient with calf-limited DVT and therefore find ultrasound adequate. Other clinicians feel that calf vein thrombosis can propagate over time to involve the larger, more proximal veins and therefore consider the definitive exclusion of calf thrombosis to be important, even if the larger veins are clear. To say the least, this point remains controversial.

The difficulty with the pelvic veins is also of some concern. Certainly thrombus localised to the pelvic veins with normal femoral and popliteal veins is uncommon. It does occur, however, and for this reason alone, I would advocate the use of venography if there was remaining clinical suspicion of a DVT following normal Doppler examination of the femoral and popliteal veins.

D. PULMONARY EMBOLISM

1. Chest X-ray

- The chest X-ray signs of pulmonary embolism are highly variable and unreliable.
- The main uses of chest X-ray are: (a) to exclude other conditions (e.g. pneumonia); (b) to aid in the interpretation of ventilation/perfusion lung scans.

(ii) clot may be seen as echogenic material in the vessel lumen;
(iii) lack of normal Doppler signal;
(iv) lack of augmentation of Doppler signal with calf compression.

2. Venography (*Fig. 13.5*)

- Filling defects within contrast-filled vessels.
- Non-filling of occluded deep veins.

Venography of the lower limb in the assessment of DVT has been largely replaced by ultrasound. Ultrasound, however, has two limitations:
(i)   the calf veins are imaged with difficulty, even with colour, and as such ultrasound does not reliably exclude DVT within these vessels in all cases;
(ii) the pelvic veins are imaged with difficulty.

2. Ventilation/perfusion lung scan (*Fig. 13.6*).

- Ventilation phase: ^{99m}Tc-DTPA aerosol.
- Perfusion phase: ^{99m}Tc-MAA (macroaggregated albumen).
- Screening test of choice.
- Pulmonary embolism is indicated by the presence of mismatched defects, i.e. defects present on the perfusion phase not matched on the ventilation phase.
- Following correlation with a chest X-ray, scans are usually graded as indicating low, intermediate, or high probability of pulmonary embolism.

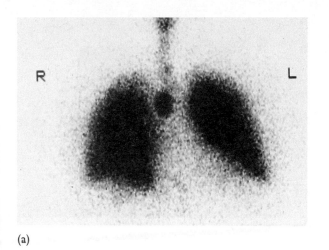
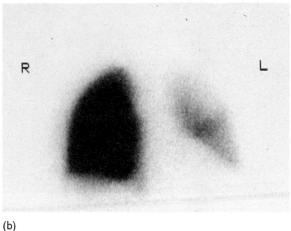

(a)   (b)

Fig. 13.6   Pulmonary embolism – ventilation/perfusion lung scan
a) Ventilation phase
Note homogeneous distribution of inhaled radio-pharmaceutical.
b) Perfusion phase
There is decreased perfusion of the left lung. Blood flow to the right lung is normal. This appearance was due to a large embolus in the left pulmonary artery.

- Unfortunately, up to 50% of ventilation/perfusion scans will be reported as showing intermediate probability, requiring either a reassessment of the clinical situation or pulmonary angiography.

3. Pulmonary angiography

- Indicated when the ventilation/perfusion scan is equivocal, i.e. shows an intermediate probability of pulmonary embolism or as a precursor to streptokinase infusion.
- Emboli show as filling defects within pulmonary artery branches with poor filling or 'cut-off' of arterial branches.

4. Interventional procedures

- Streptokinase infusion directly into affected pulmonary arteries via the angiography catheter.
- Caval filters inserted into the IVC under screening control indicated where: (a) anticoagulation is contra-indicated; (b) recurrent pulmonary embolism occurs despite adequate anticoagulation.

E. ABDOMINAL AORTIC ANEURYSM

1. Ultrasound

- Shows anatomy of aneurysm, i.e. shape, size, relation to renal arteries and aortic bifurcation.
- Thrombosis.
- Leakage.
- Other complications (e.g. hydronephrosis).
- May be difficult due to overlying bowel gas or obesity.

2. CT (*Fig. 13.7*)

- Often performed as investigation of first choice and/or where ultrasound is difficult.
- Shows anatomy of aneurysm, as above, as well as thrombus and evidence of leakage.
- Anatomical variants which may be important to know about pre-operatively (e.g. horeshoe kidney, retroaortic left renal vein).

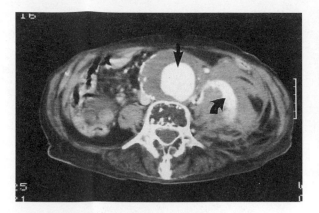

Fig. 13.7 Ruptured abdominal aortic aneurysm – CT
Note: • dilated aorta
   • contrast-filled lumen (straight arrow) surrounded by non-enhancing thrombus
   • left retroperitoneal haematoma
   • leakage of contrast indicating active haemorrhage at the time of the scan (curved arrow).

• Complicated cases (e.g. inflammatory aneurysm).
• Post-operative: assessment of grafts, aorto-duodenal fistula.
• Early work indicates that CT angiography (CTA) may also be useful in displaying a 3D image of aortic aneurysms.

3. Angiography

• Rarely required prior to surgery as CT and ultrasound usually provide adequate information.

F. AORTIC DISSECTION

1. Plain films

• Unreliable, i.e. chest X-ray is often normal in the face of significant dissection.
• Any or all of the following signs may be seen and mostly relate to the presence of mediastinal haematoma secondary to rupture of the dissection:
   (i) mediastinal widening;
   (ii) pleural fluid;
   (iii) widening of the paravertebral stripe;
   (iv) depression of the left main bronchus;

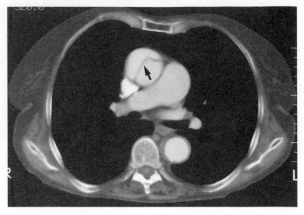

Fig. 13.8 Aortic dissection – CT
Note the intimal flap in the ascending aorta outlined by contrast in the true and false lumina (arrow).

   (v) separation of intimal calcification from the margin of the aortic outline.

2. CT scans (*Fig. 13.8*)

• Scans should be performed during the infusion of intravenous contrast (i.e. dynamic contrast CT).
• Signs are as follows:
   (i) differentiation of true from false lumen;
   (ii) intimal flap;
   (iii) mediastinal haematoma/pleural fluid indicating rupture;
   (iv) involvement of branch vessels and infarction of organs (e.g. kidneys, liver, spleen).

3. MRI (*Fig. 13.9*)

• Excellent contrast between flowing blood and soft tissue allows good delineation of true and false lumina.
• Ability to image in sagittal and oblique planes allows good assessment of intimal flap and extent of dissection.

4. Angiography

• May be required for better definition prior to surgery.

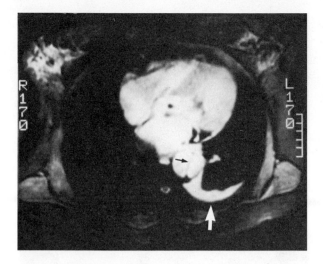

Fig. 13.9   Aortic dissection – MRI
Note: • intimal flap in the descending aorta outlined by
         high signal blood in the true and false lumina
         (black arrow).
       • left haemothorax (white arrow).

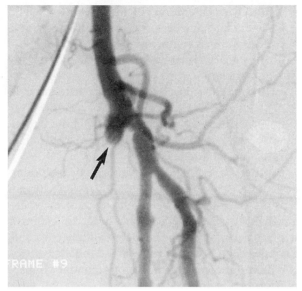

Fig. 13.10   Occluded superficial femoral artery –
angiogram
Note: • occlusion of the superficial femoral artery
         (arrow)
       • large branches of the profunda femoris artery
         supplying blood to the lower limb.

G. PERIPHERAL ARTERIAL DISEASE (I.E. ASSESSMENT FOR CLAUDICATION AND ISCHAEMIA)

1. Angiography (*Fig. 13.10*)

- Remains the investigation of choice for delineating stenoses and occlusions, atheroma, and collateral flow.
- May be used in conjunction with interventional procedures:
  (i)   angioplasty;
  (ii) placement of endovascular stents;
  (iii) streptokinase infusion for acute thrombo-embolism causing arterial obstruction.

2. Ultrasound

- Doppler ultrasound with colour can be used to localise stenoses and diagnose arterial obstruction.
- Intravascular ultrasound.

3. MR angiography (MRA)

- Early experience indicates that MRA may eventually replace angiography in the diagnosis of peripheral arterial disease.
- Angiography will still be used in association with interventional procedures.

H. HYPERTENSION

The great majority of hypertensive patients have essential hypertension. The clinical challenge is to identify the small percentage of patients with secondary hypertension and to delineate any treatable lesions. All hypertensive patients should have a chest X-ray for the following reasons:

- Diagnosis of cardiovascular complications (e.g. cardiac enlargement, aortic valve calcification, cardiac failure).
- To establish a baseline for monitoring of future changes or complications such as aortic dissection.

- Rarely, coarctation of the aorta may be detected; signs of aortic coarctation on chest X-ray are as follows:
  (i) cardiac enlargement, especially left ventricle;
  (ii) indentation of contour of aortic knuckle giving the configuration of a figure '3';
  (iii) bilateral rib notching involving the undersurface of ribs 3–8 due to enlarged intercostal arteries.

Further investigation is indicated in young patients, i.e. less than 40 years old, where hypertension is severe or malignant in nature; where antihypertensive medication fails to control hypertension; or in the presence of certain clinical signs (e.g. bruit heard over the renal arteries).

The more common causes of secondary hypertension are as follows:
(a) *Renal*
  - Renal artery stenosis.
  - Diseases leading to renal failure.
(b) *Vascular*
  - Coarctation of the aorta.
(c) *Endocrine*
  - Phaeochromocytoma.
  - Conn's syndrome (i.e. primary hyperaldosteronism).
  - Cushing's syndrome.

Initial investigations usually consist of:
(i) biochemical testing of renal function and endocrine studies;
(ii) screening tests for renal artery stenosis.

Screening tests for renal artery stenosis and renal disease are as follows:

1. Ultrasound

- Measurement of renal size.
- Assessment of renal morphology.
- Doppler examination of renal arteries: stenosis indicated by an increase in blood flow velocity above a certain level.
- Major limitation is difficulty of imaging renal arteries due to:
  (i) overlying bowel gas;
  (ii) obesity;
  (iii) presence of multiple, aberrant arteries.
- These problems may be overcome by direct Doppler examination of flow characteris-

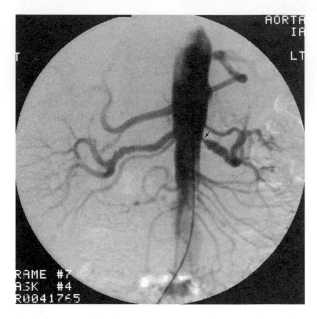

Fig. 13.11   Renal artery stenosis – angiogram
This case demonstrates the two principal types of renal artery lesion. There is a tight localised stenosis at the origin of the left renal artery due to atheroma (arrow). Note also the irregular, beaded appearance of both renal arteries due to fibromuscular hyperplasia.

tics of small arteries within the kidneys; early results of research in this area are promising.

2. Scintigraphy

- ^{99m}Tc-DTPA.
- The use of intravenous captopril increases the accuracy of the study.
- Renal blood flow.
- Renal size and outline.
- Differential function.
- Drainage of collecting systems.

Note that this is a screening test only and renal artery morphology is not assessed.

Depending on the results of either or both of the above tests, more specific imaging for renal artery stenosis may be performed, as below:

(a) Renal angiogram (*Fig. 13.11*)

- Aortogram to delineate renal arteries including aberrent vessels.
- Selective injection of renal arteries.

- Two types of lesion found:
  (i) *atheroma*: localised narrowing of the renal artery origin;
  (ii) *fibromuscular hyperplasia*: the renal artery has an irregular beaded appearance.
- These two lesions may co-exist in the same patient.

(b) Renal vein renins:

- Via the femoral vein catheters are positioned in the renal veins; blood samples are taken from each renal vein to assess renin levels.
- Selective sampling from smaller branches may also be performed.
- A positive renal vein renin study indicates a favourable outcome from surgery or interventional radiology.

(c) Angioplasty:

- As for peripheral arteries angioplasty, i.e. dilatation of the artery with a balloon catheter, can be performed on renal arteries.

Endocrine causes as indicated by clinical signs and symptoms as well as results of biochemical tests, may be outlined as follows:

(a) Phaeochromocytoma:

(i) CT
  - Concentrates initially on the adrenals with further studies of the remainder of the abdomen if no tumour is found.
(ii) Scintigraphy
  - ^{99m}Tc-MIBG.
  - MIBG (metaiodobenzylguanidine) is a noradrenaline analogue.
  - Localisation of phaeochromocytoma anywhere in the body.

(b) Primary hyperaldosteronism:

(i) CT
  - Use of fine sections and intravenous contrast gives optimal visualisation of the adrenal glands.
(ii) Adrenal vein sampling
  - Via the femoral veins, fine catheters may be placed within the adrenal veins for the purpose of selective venous sampling and hence diagnosis and localisation of the source of hyperaldosteronism.
  - Differentiate unilateral tumour, i.e. Conn's tumour from bilateral hyperplasia.

(c) Cushing's disease

(i) CT of adrenal glands.
(ii) MRI of pituitary fossa.

Further Reading

1. Bernard SA, Jones BM, Stuckey JG. Pulmonary angiography in a non-teaching hospital over a 12-year period. *MJA* 1992;**157**:589–592.
2. Cigarroa JE, Isselbacher EM, DeSanctis RW, Eagle KA. Medical progress. Diagnostic imaging in the evaluation of suspected aortic dissection; old standards and new directions. *AJR* 1993;**161**:485–493.
3. Editorial: Venous thrombosis and thromboembolism. *Clinical Radiology* 1990;**41**:77–80.
4. Editorial: Ventilation/perfusion scan in pulmonary embolism: 'The emperor is incompletely attired'. *JAMA* 1990;**263**:2794–2795.
5. McGarth BP, Clarke K. Renal artery stenosis: current diagnosis and treatment. *MJA* 1993;**158**:343–345.
6. Middleton WD. Doppler US evaluation of renal artery stenosis: past, present and future. *Radiology* 1992;**184**:307–308.
7. Murphy P, Wilde P. Non-invasive imaging of the cardiac patient. *Current Imaging* 1990;**2**:42–48.
8. Raymond HW, Zwiebel WJ, Harnsberger HR (eds). Advances in cardiac imaging. *Seminars in Ultrasound, CT and MR* 1991;**12**:1.
9. Wilde P. *Doppler Echocardiography: An Illustrated Clinical Guide*. Churchill Livingstone, 1989.

14
Respiratory system

A. CT
B. High-resolution CT (HRCT)
C. Scintigraphy
D. Ultrasound
E. Imaging of sinus disease

Virtually all symptoms and clinical situations related to the respiratory system will be investigated primarily by chest X-ray. Interpretation of chest X-rays has been outlined in Chapter 4. Therefore, here I briefly outline the role of the main imaging modalities in respiratory disease, in general, rather than considering specific symptoms, as elsewhere.

A. CT

CT is the investigation of choice for the following.

- Mediastinal mass.
    (i) accurate localisation;
    (ii) internal contents of mass (e.g. fat, air, fluid, calcification);
    (iii) displacement/invasion of adjacent structures (e.g. great vessels, heart, trachea, oesophagus, vertebral column, chest wall).
- Hilar mass (*Fig. 14.1*)
    (i) greater sensitivity than plain films for the presence of hilar lymphadenopathy;
    (ii) greater specificity in differentiating lymphadenopathy or hilar mass from enlarged pulmonary arteries.

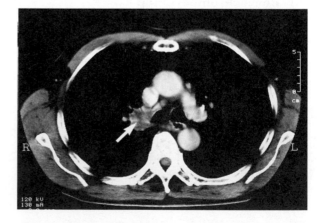

Fig. 14.1   Bronchogenic carcinoma – CT
Note: • mass at the right hilum (arrow)
       • non-enhancement of the mass compared with densely enhanced contrast-filled mediastinal blood vessels, i.e. SVC, aorta, left pulmonary artery.

- Staging of bronchogenic carcinoma, lymphoma, and other malignancies:
  - (i) greater sensitivity than plain films for the presence of mediastinal or hilar lymphadenopathy;
  - (ii) greater sensitivity for complications such as chest wall or mediastinal invasion, cavitation.
- Detection of pulmonary metastases:
  - (i) CT has greater sensitivity than plain films for the detection of small pulmonary lesions, including metastases;
  - (ii) this is particularly so in areas of the lung seen poorly on CXR (e.g. the apices, posterior segments of the lower lobes, medial areas obscured by the hila).
- Characterisation of a pulmonary mass seen on CXR:
  - (i) more accurate than plain films for the presence of calcification;
  - (ii) other factors also well assessed by CT include: cavitation, relation of a mass to chest wall/mediastinum;
  - (iii) iv contrast may help to identify aberrant vessels/arterio-venous malformations.
- Demonstration of mediastinal vasculature:
  - (i) thoracic aortic aneurysm;
  - (ii) aortic dissection;
  - (iii) SVC compression/invasion by tumour;
  - (iv) vascular anomalies which may cause odd shadows on CXR (e.g. azygos continuation of IVC, partial anomalous pulmonary venous drainage).
- Trauma:
  - (i) exclusion of mediastinal haematoma in a haemodynamically stable patient with a widened mediastinum on CXR following chest trauma;
  - (ii) haemodynamically unstable patients should go immediately to angiography or operating theatre.
- Characterisation of pleural disease:
  - (i) CT gives excellent delineation of pleural abnormalities which may produce confusing appearances on CXR;
  - (ii) pleural masses, fluid collections, calcification, and tumour such as mesothelioma are well shown, as are complications such as rib destruction, mediastinal invasion, and lymphadenopathy.

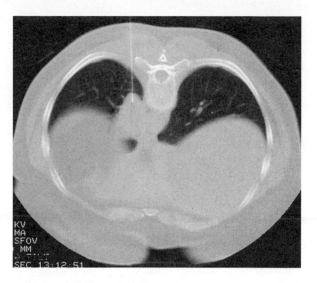

Fig. 14.2 CT-guided biopsy
Note placement of a biopsy needle into a mass in the left lower lobe. Cytology showed a squamous cell carcinoma.

- Guidance of percutaneous biopsy/drainage procedures:
  - (i) especially useful for peripheral lesions not amenable to biopsy via bronchoscope (*Fig. 14.2*).

B. HIGH-RESOLUTION CT (HRCT)

High-resolution CT is a technique used in the assessment of disorders of the lungs. Conventional CT of the chest uses sections 5–10 mm in thickness spaced 10 mm apart. The high-resolution technique uses much thinner sections of around 1 mm thickness, spaced 10–15 mm apart. The thinner sections show much greater lung detail. Intravenous contrast is not used and the mediastinal and chest wall structures are less well seen than with conventional chest CT. High-resolution CT is useful in the following.

1. Bronchiectasis (*Fig. 14.3*)

- HRCT has all but replaced bronchography in the assessment of bronchiectasis.

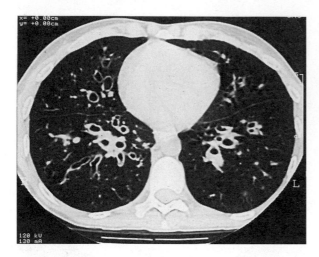

Fig. 14.3   Bronchiectasis – HRCT
There are dilated bronchi with thickened walls in the right middle lobe and both lower lobes.

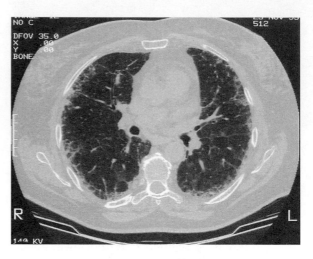

Fig. 14.4   Interstitial pneumonia (fibrosing alveolitis) – HRCT
Note the typical distribution of peripheral subpleural fibrosis. Compare this appearance with more normal looking central lung tissue.

- As well as showing dilated bronchi, HRCT accurately shows the anatomical distribution of changes, in addition to complications such as scarring, collapse, consolidation, and mucous plugging.

2.   Interstitial lung disease (*Fig. 14.4*)

- HRCT is more sensitive and specific than plain films in the diagnosis of many interstitial lung diseases.
- Sarcoidosis, interstitial pneumonia (fibrosing alveolitis), lymphangitis carcinomatosa, and histiocytosis-X are examples of disorders that have specific appearances on HRCT, often obviating the need for biopsy in these patients.
- Where biopsy is felt necessary, HRCT may aid in guiding the operator to the most favourable biopsy site.

3.   Atypical infections

- HRCT provides diagnosis of many atypical infections earlier and with greater specificity than plain CXR.
- Examples include: pneumocystis carinii, aspergillosis, and mycobacterium avium intracellulare, infections which occur in immunocompromised patients, including those with AIDS.
- As well as diagnosis, HRCT may be useful for monitoring disease progress and response to therapy.

4.   Normal CXR in symptomatic patients

- HRCT has a definite role in the assessment of patients with an apparently normal CXR, despite the clinical indications of respiratory disease, including dyspnoea, chest pain, haemoptysis, abnormal pulmonary function tests.

C. SCINTIGRAPHY

A number of examples exist of the use of scintigraphy in the assessment of disorders of the respiratory system.

1.   Pulmonary embolism

- Ventilation/perfusion lung scan.

2.   Early infection

- Gallium-67 (^{67}Ga).

- May be used in the detection of early infection.
- The most common example in clinical use would be in the detection of early pneumocystis carinii infection in AIDS patients: increased lung uptake of ^{67}Ga may be seen prior to the appearance of CXR changes.

D. ULTRASOUND

1. Echocardiography

The chief application for ultrasound in the chest is in echocardiography. Visualisation of the heart may be difficult in emphysematous patients where the heart is covered by overexpanded lung. This difficulty is overcome with the use of transoesophageal probes.

2. Pleural fluid

Ultrasound is useful for the confirmation of pleural effusion suspected on CXR. Ultrasound is also very useful for guidance of drainage of small pleural fluid collections.

E. IMAGING OF SINUS DISEASE

1. Sinus X-rays

- At best, a crude screening test.
- Fluid levels in sinuses indicate acute sinusitis.
- Mucosal thickening/total opacification indicate 'sinusitis' which may be acute, chronic, or allergic.
- No information on sinus ostia.
- Not accurate for underlying bony abnormalities.

2. Coronal CT of the paranasal sinuses

- Imaging investigation of choice in the diagnosis and assessment of sinus diseases, especially in the pre-operative assessment of chronic sinusitis.

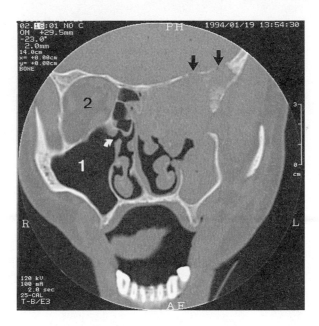

Fig. 14.5   Ethmoid sinus carcinoma – coronal CT
Note:
- soft tissue mass filling left ethmoid and maxillary sinuses
- invasion of the left orbit
- bone destruction indicating a malignant process (straight arrows)
- normal structures on the right: maxillary sinus (1), maxillary ostium (curved arrow), orbit (2).

- The following factors are assessed by CT prior to functional endoscopic sinus surgery:
  - (i) distribution and nature of sinus disease: fluid levels, mucosal thickening, polyps;
  - (ii) state of maxillary ostia;
  - (iii) underlying anatomical variants (e.g. nasal septum deviation, concha bullosa, configuration of osteo-infundibular complexes, etc.);
  - (iv) evidence of sinus tumour: soft tissue mass with bone destruction (*Fig. 14.5*);
  - (v) mucocele formation: soft tissue mass with sinus expansion.

Further Reading

1. Brown LR, Aughenbaugh GL. Masses of the anterior mediastinum: CT and MR imaging. *AJR* 1991;**157**:1171–1180.

2.   Goddard P, Cook P, Hartnell G, Troughton A, Kinsella D. Magnetic resonance imaging of the thorax. *Current Imaging* 1989;**1**:175–180.

3.   McLoud TC, Flower CDR. Imaging the pleura: sonography, CT, and MR imaging. *AJR* 1991;**156**:1145–1153.

4.   Mafee MF. Endoscopic sinus surgery: role of the radiologist. *AJNR* 1991;**12**:855–860.

5.   Mafee MF, Chow JM, Meyers R. Functional endoscopic sinus surgery: anatomy, CT screening, indications, and complications. *AJR* 1993;**160**:735–744.

6.   Swensen SJ, Aughenbaugh GL, Douglas WW, Myers JL. High-resolution CT of the lungs: findings in various pulmonary diseases. *AJR* 1992;**158**:971–979.

7.   Webb RW, Muller NL, Naidich DP. *High-Resolution CT of the Lung*. Raven Press, 1992.

8.   Yousem DM. Imaging of sinonasal inflammatory disease. *Radiology* 1993;**188**:303–314.

15
Gastrointestinal tract

A. Dysphagia
B. Acute cholecystitis
C. Acute pancreatitis
D. Inflammatory bowel disease
E. Gastrointestinal bleeding
F. Meckel's diverticulum
G. Abdominal trauma
H. Suspected abdominal abscess
I. Jaundice
J. Suspected liver mass

A DYSPHAGIA

Barium swallow

- Simplest, cheapest, and most effective screening test.
- Often sufficient for diagnosis or may provide a guide to further procedures or imaging as required, e.g. endoscopic assessment and biopsy of a stricture.
- Commonly encountered conditions and findings are as follows.
1. Pharyngeal pouch (Zenker's diverticulum):
   - Projects posteriorly and to the left in the neck above the cricopharyngeus muscle.
2. Achalasia:
   - Dilated oesophagus with poor peristalsis and a smoothly tapered lower end.
   - Chest X-ray may show an absent gastric air bubble and a fluid level in the mediastinum.
3. Hiatus hernia
   - Range in size from a small hernia to thoracic stomach, i.e. the entire stomach lying within the thorax.
   - Chest X-ray may show an apparent mass containing a fluid level posterior to the heart.
4. Oesophageal diverticulae:
   - Usually project antero-laterally and most common between the level of the tracheal bifurcation and the diaphragm.
5. Reflux oesophagitis:
   - Erosions and ulcers seen as mucosal defects which retain barium.
   - Chronic reflux may cause a peptic stricture which usually has smooth, tapering edges.
6. Carcinoma of the oesophagus:
   - Range of appearances depending on tumour size and growth pattern.
   - Early mucosal irregularity and ulceration.
   - Later irregular stricture formation.
   - May also see a mass or sinus/fistula formation.
   - For further imaging as indicated for tumour staging see Chapter 22.
7. Functional oesophageal disorders:
   - A wide range of functional oesophageal disorders are seen in elderly patients presenting with dysphagia.

- A range of appearances is seen from a dilated oesophagus with poor peristalsis to an irregular, corkscrew outline due to sustained contractions of the oesophageal wall.
8. Functional swallowing disorders:
   - Swallowing and feeding problems due to neuromuscular incoordination of the oral cavity or pharynx are common in the elderly and due to a wide range of CNS problems, most commonly CVA, head injury, and degenerative CNS disorders.
   - Lateral films are taken of the oral cavity, pharynx, and upper oesophagus during swallowing; the procedure is usually recorded on video for later close perusal.

B. ACUTE CHOLECYSTITIS

I. Ultrasound (*Fig. 15.1*)

- Investigation of choice.
- Gallstones: hyperechoic lesions with distal acoustic shadowing; may be mobile or impacted in the gallbladder neck and associated with gallbladder distension.

- Thickening of the gall-bladder wall with a surrounding hypoechoic layer due to oedema.
- Localised tenderness to direct pressure with the ultrasound probe.

2. Scintigraphy

- HIDA scan: ^{99m}Tc labelled iminodiacetic acid (IDA) compounds; the 'H' stands for hepatobiliary.
- Used in cases where the clinical signs and/or ultrasound examination are equivocal.
- Acute cholecystitis: non-visualisation of the gallbladder with good visualisation of the common bile duct and duodenum 1 hour after injection.

C. ACUTE PANCREATITIS

I. CT scan (*Fig. 15.2*)

- Investigation of choice.
- Roles:
  (i) confirm the diagnosis;

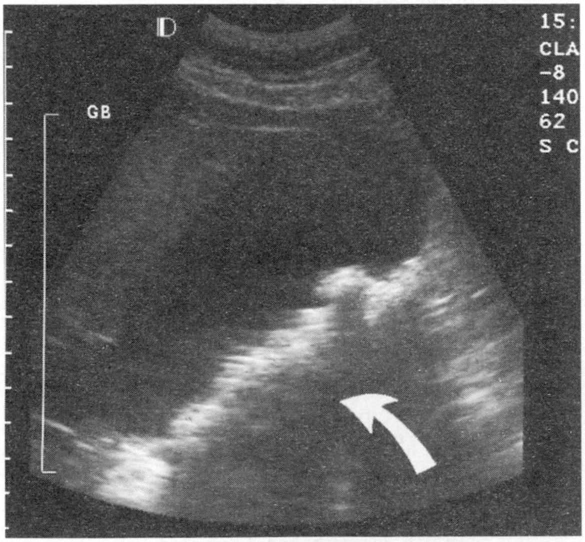

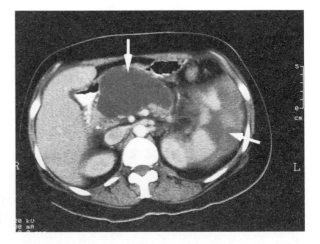

Fig. 15.1   Gallstones – ultrasound
Note: • multiple gallstones seen as hyperechoic structures forming a layer within the gallbladder
      • prominent acoustic shadow (arrow).

Fig. 15.2   Pancreatitis – CT
Note: • pancreatic pseudocyst seen as a low-attenuation fluid-filled structure lying posterior to the stomach in the neck and body of the pancreas (upper arrow).
      • fluid around the lower pole of the spleen (arrow on right).

(ii) identify necrotic pancreatic tissue;

(iii) diagnose complications;

(iv) guide interventional procedures (e.g. abscess or pseudocyst drainage).

- Signs of acute pancreatitis:
  (i) diffuse or focal gland enlargement with decreased attenuation and indistinct gland margins;
  (ii) necrotic tissue fails to enhance with intravenous contrast;
  (iii) thickening of surrounding fascial planes, e.g. the left pararenal fascia and increased density of surrounding fat due to inflammatory change.

- Complications:
  (i) fluid collections: most commonly related to the pancreas itself, lesser sac, left paranephric space;
  (ii) phlegmon: irregular mass spreading along fascial planes;
  (iii) pseudocyst: fluid-filled lesion with a well-defined wall;
  (iv) abscess: fluid-filled lesion with poorly-defined, irregular wall.

2. Ultrasound

- Often difficult in the acute situation owing to overlying dilated bowel loops.
- Less definition of fascial planes than CT.
- Fluid collections, phlegmon, pseudocyst, and abscess may be seen.

D. INFLAMMATORY BOWEL DISEASE

1. Plain films

- Should be performed in acute presentations to diagnose toxic megacolon in which case barium studies are contraindicated.
- Signs of toxic megacolon:
  (i) markedly dilated segment of bowel, usually transverse colon to greater than 8.0 cm diameter;
  (ii) often complicated by perforation and peritonitis.
- Signs of acute colitis:
  (i) bowel wall thickening;

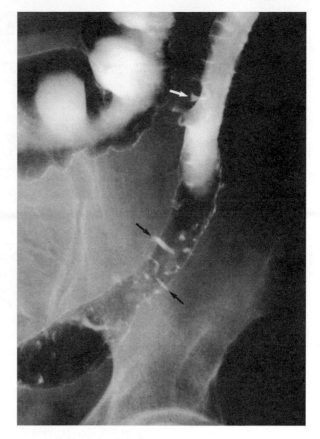

Fig. 15.3 Crohn's disease – barium enema
Note deep 'rose thorn' type ulceration involving the descending colon (arrows).

(ii) absent haustral markings;

(iii) gasless colon.

2. Barium studies

(a) Crohn's disease (*Figs. 15.3* and *15.4*)

- Small bowel enema and barium enema.
- 'Skip' lesions, i.e. diseased segments separated by normal appearing bowel.
- Ulcers, strictures, fistulae and sinuses, bowel wall thickening.
- 'Cobblestone' appearance due to fissures of barium separating islands of intact mucosa.
- Abscesses may cause displacement of bowel loops, especially in the right iliac fossa.

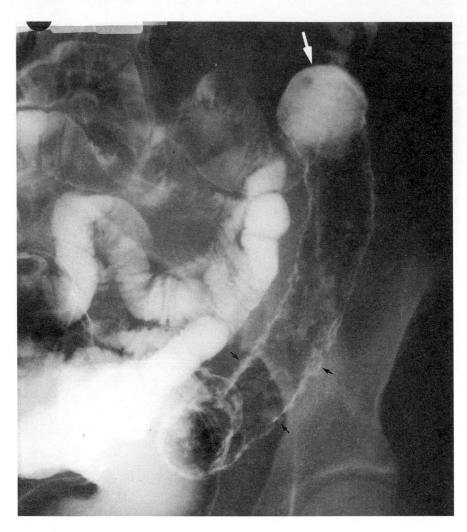

Fig. 15.4 Recurrent Crohn's disease – barium enema
Note:
- previous partial colectomy with small bowel anastomosed to splenic flexure (white arrow)
- abnormal sigmoid and descending colon with loss of haustra and deep ulceration (black arrows)
- sparing of the rectum.

(b)   Ulcerative colits (*Fig. 15.5*)

- Barium enema.
- Retrograde involvement of the large bowel, including the rectum, with no skip lesions.
- *Early*: fine ulceration.
- *Late*: loss of haustral markings with shortening and narrowing of the large bowel.
- Pseudopolyp formation due to post-inflammatory granulation tissue and fibrosis.

E. GASTROINTESTINAL BLEEDING

Endoscopy is the primary investigation of choice for acute upper and lower gastrointestinal bleeding. In a proportion of patients, however, endoscopy will fail to either diagnose the cause of bleeding or achieve haemostasis. In these patients a variety of radiological methods may be used.

I. Angiography

- Performed for two reasons: to locate a bleeding point; and to achieve haemostasis by:
    (i) infusion of vasoconstrictors (vasopressin);
    (ii) embolisation.
- Selective injection of coeliac axis, superior mesenteric artery, and inferior mesenteric artery.

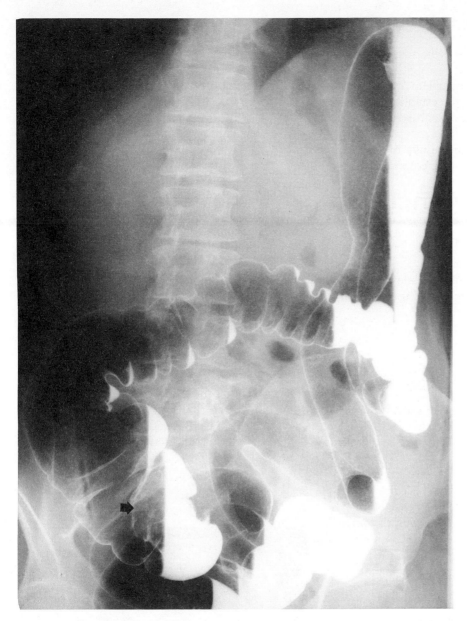

Fig. 15.5 Ulcerative colitis –
barium enema
Note:
- loss of normal haustra in
  the left colon
- pattern of fine mucosal
  ulceration giving the bowel
  a 'shaggy' outline
- this case is complicated by
  a carcinoma, seen as a
  mass in the caecum
  (arrow).

- Acute bleeding at a rate of 0.5 ml per minute or greater will be shown by leakage of contrast into the bowel lumen.
- Diverticular disease is the most common cause of acute lower gastrointestinal bleeding in elderly patients: contrast may be seen filling a diverticulum.
- Vascular disorders may also be diagnosed, of which the most common is angiodysplasia:
  (i)   occurs in elderly patients;
  (ii) most common in the ascending colon;
  (iii) small nest of irregular vessels with early, persistent filling of a draining vein.

2. Scintigraphy

- ^{99m}Tc labelled red blood cells.
- More sensitive than angiography, i.e. a lower rate of haemorrhage of the order of

0.1 ml per minute is required to give a positive test.

- Less anatomically specific than angiography.
- Usually used in a complementary role to angiography, i.e. to establish whether acute haemorrhage is occurring prior to angiography.
- Surgery based on the results of scintigraphy alone would not be recommended.

F. MECKEL'S DIVERTICULUM

I. Small bowel enema

- Investigation of choice.
- Meckel's diverticulum shows as a contrast-filled pouch arising from the distal small bowel.

2. Scintigraphy

- ^{99m}Tc, i.e. free technetium or pertechnetate.
- Accuracy quite low, so should be used if small bowel enema is equivocal.
- Pertechnetate is taken up by gastric mucosa.
- A positive test occurs where the diverticulum contains aberrant gastric mucosa and shows as a small, localised area of increased activity in the lower abdomen.

G. ABDOMINAL TRAUMA

I. Plain films

- Plain-film findings are unreliable, and in suspected solid organ damage CT is the investigation of choice.
- Plain-film findings in abdominal trauma include:
  (i) free gas in perforation of the gastrointestinal tract;
  (ii) free gas from ruptured duodenum as occurs classically in seat-belt injuries may collect in the retroperitoneal space and therefore outline the psoas margin;
  (iii) intraperitoneal fluid: general greyness

of the abdomen; and displacement of bowel loops;
  (iv) bony lesions: rib fractures, spinal fractures, and pelvic fractures;
  (v) chest changes: pleural effusion, lower lobe collapse, ruptured diaphragm, and free gas beneath the diaphragm.

2. CT

- CT with intravenous contrast is the imaging investigation of choice for severe abdominal trauma.
- Peritoneal fluid/fluid collections: blood appears as low-density material in dependent parts of the peritoneal cavity (i.e. the pelvis, hepatorenal fossa, paracolic gutters).
- Splenic trauma:
  (i) altered organ contour and density;
  (ii) lacerations appear as hypodense lines separating more dense splenic fragments (*Fig. 15.6*).
- Hepatic trauma:
  (i) intrahepatic haematomas are well localised by CT and may be of increased or decreased attenuation.
  (ii) lacerations appear as hypodense lines in the liver substance.

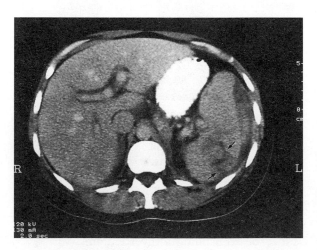

Fig. 15.6   Splenic rupture – CT
Note: • subcapsular haematoma
      • lacerations seen as low-attenuation lines through the spleen (arrows).

3. Ultrasound

- May be difficult in the traumatised patient owing to dilated bowel loops, wound dressings, etc.
- Will show free fluid, fluid collections, hepatic and splenic trauma.
- Good technique for follow-up of patients who have been managed conservatively.

4. Angiography

- Limited role in abdominal trauma.
- Occasionally used to localise bleeding and treat with embolisation.

H. SUSPECTED ABDOMINAL ABSCESS

I. Ultrasound

- Primary investigation of choice.
- An abscess is seen as an anechoic fluid collection with an irregular, ill-defined wall.
- Ultrasound is especially sensitive to subdiaphragmatic, subhepatic, and pelvic collections.

2. CT

- Excellent modality, especially where ultrasound is unhelpful.
- The bowel must be opacified with oral contrast as non-opacified bowel loops may mimic fluid collections.
- Both ultrasound and CT may be used to guide aspiration and drainage placement.

3. Scintigraphy

- Indium-111 or ^{99m}Tc-HMPAO (hexamethylpropyleneamine oxime) labelled white blood cells or gallium-67 (^{67}Ga).
- Used in difficult cases where clinical suspicion of an abscess is high but ultrasound and CT are negative.
- An abscess shows as a localised area of increased activity.

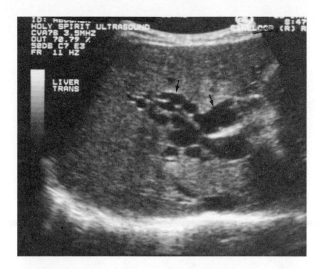

Fig. 15.7 Dilated bile ducts – ultrasound
Dilated intrahepatic bile ducts seen as branching fluid-filled structures in the liver (arrows).

I. JAUNDICE

I. Ultrasound

- Initial investigation of choice in most cases.
- Differentiates obstructive from non-obstructive jaundice, i.e. distinguishes dilated from non-dilated bile ducts.
- Common bile duct measurements:
  (i) normal < 6 mm;
  (ii) equivocal 6–8 mm;
  (iii) dilated > 8 mm.
- Dilated intrahepatic ducts show a branching pattern radiating from the porta, often best seen in the left hepatic lobe (*Fig. 15.7*).
- When the bile ducts are dilated, the site and cause of obstruction can be defined in only about 25% of cases as the lower common bile duct is often obscured by overlying intestinal gas.
- In the absence of bile duct dilatation, ultrasound may identify diffuse or focal liver diseases (e.g. cirrhosis, fatty infiltration, masses, metastases).
- Ultrasound can be used to guide biopsy of focal or diffuse liver abnormalities.

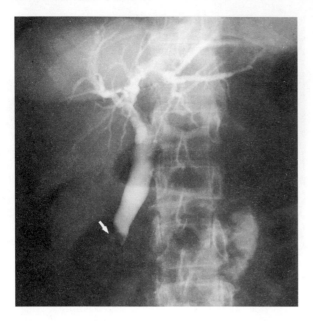

Fig. 15.8 Carcinoma of the ampulla of vater – ERCP
Dilated common bile duct with an irregular stricture at its
lower end (arrow).

2.   ERCP (*Fig. 15.8*)

- Usually performed after ultrasound shows dilated bile ducts.
- Defines site and nature of obstruction.
- May be combined with sphincterotomy, basket stone extraction, stent insertion.
- Stones show as filling defects: single/ multiple; mobile/impacted; round/faceted.
- Carcinoma of the pancreas shows as a smoothly tapering stricture of the lower end of the common bile duct.

3.   PTC

- Used in obstructive jaundice where:
  (i) ERCP has failed to outline the duct system or define the obstructing lesion;
  (ii) ultrasound or CT suggest a high obstructing lesion in which case PTC is often the preferred procedure.

4.   CT

- Biliary dilatation is seen as a low-attenuation branching pattern in the liver.

- Dilated common bile duct is also identified.
- As with ultrasound, in the absence of bile duct dilatation, diffuse or focal liver lesions may be seen as a cause for jaundice.

5.   Scintigraphy

- ^{99m}Tc-IDA (HIDA scan).
- Limited role in jaundice due to impaired excretion and hence poor visualisation of the duct system where serum bilirubin is elevated.
- Findings may be as follows:
  (i) failure of liver uptake: severe liver dysfunction;
  (ii) normal liver uptake, non-visualisation of bile ducts: cholestasis or high obstruction;
  (iii) visualisation of bile ducts, non-visualisation of duodenum: low biliary obstruction.

J.   SUSPECTED LIVER MASS

1.   CT with intravenous contrast

- CT with injection of intravenous contrast is the imaging modality of choice in the assessment of most liver masses.
- Helical scanning allows examination of the liver during optimal concentration of contrast medium.
- The roles of CT in assessment of liver masses are as follows:
  (i)   anatomical localisation
  (ii) define margins of the lesion;
  (iii) specific information on contents (e.g. calcification, gas, fluid, fat);
  (iv) identify multiple lesions;
  (v)   guidance of biopsy or abscess drainage.

2.   Ultrasound (*Fig. 15.9*)

- Usually complementary to CT, i.e. provides further characterisation of certain lesions.

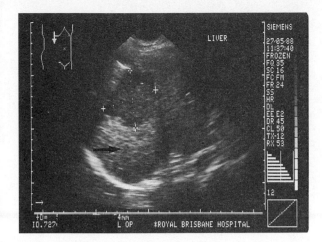

Fig. 15.9 Liver abscess – ultrasound
Note: • hypoechoic lesion in the right lobe of the liver
      • irregular wall
      • acoustic enhancement indicating that the lesion contains fluid (arrow).

- In some centres will be the primary investigation of choice for suspected liver mass.
- As with CT, ultrasound provides good anatomical localisation, as well as information on the internal structure and margins of a mass.

3. Scintigraphy

- ^{99m}Tc-colloid.
- Usually a complementary role to CT and ultrasound.
- Lesions larger than 1.0 cm can be seen.

- Especially useful for the diaphragmatic surface of the liver which may be difficult to image with the other techniques.

4. Angiography

- More often used for liver masses than for masses in other organs.
- Two main roles: to outline the arterial supply of a tumour pre-operatively, as well as tumour relationship to the portal vein (hepatocellular carcinoma may invade the portal vein) and the IVC, i.e. a surgical 'roadmap'; and CT arterial portography (see Chapter 7).

Further Reading

1. Bluemke DA, Fishman EK. Spiral CT of the liver. *AJR* 1993;**160**:787–792.
2. Dixon PM, Nolan DJ. The diagnosis of Meckel's diverticulum: a continuing challenge. *Clinical Radiology* 1987;**38**:615–619.
3. Mendelson RM. The role of endoscopic ultrasonography in the upper gastrointestinal tract. *Australasian Radiology* 1993;**37**:349–359.
4. Ott DJ, Pikna LA. Clinical and videofluoroscopic evaluation of swallowing disorders. *AJR* 1993;**161**: 507–513.
5. Scatamacchia SA, Raptopoulos V, Fink MP, Silva WE. Splenic trauma in adults: impact of CT grading on management. *Radiology* 1989;**171**:725–729.
6. Stevenson GW. Radiology of gastro-oesophageal reflux. *Clinical Radiology* 1989;**40**:119–121.
7. Zuckerman DA, Bocchini TP, Birnbaum EH. Massive hemorrhage in the lower gastrointestinal tract in adults: diagnostic imaging and intervention. *AJR* 1993;**161**:703–711.

16
Urinary tract

A.   Renal mass
B.   Painless haematuria
C.   Renal colic
D.   Renal trauma
E.   Trauma to the bladder and urethra
F.   Prostatism

A. RENAL MASS

I. Ultrasound (*Fig. 16.1*)

- Reliable, safe, and cheap initial screening modality of choice for a renal mass suspected clinically or found on IVP during investigation for haematuria.
- Differentiates a simple cyst from either a complicated cyst or a solid mass.
- Criteria of simple cyst on ultrasound:
  (i) anechoic fluid contents;
  (ii) well-defined thin echogenic wall;
  (iii) distal acoustic enhancement.
- Any renal lesion not fitting the above criteria for a simple cyst requires further assessment.
- Complicated cyst refers to:
  (i) a cyst containing internal echoes which may be due to infection or haemorrhage;
  (ii) a cyst containing soft tissue septae;
  (iii) a cyst associated with a soft tissue mass.

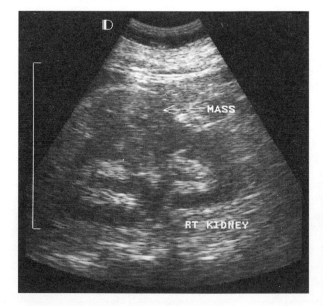

Fig. 16.1   Renal cell carcinoma – ultrasound
Note: • oval-shaped kidney with hypoechoic cortex and hyperechoic medulla
      • solid mass arising from the lateral aspect of the kidney.

- A solid mass may show:
  (i)   hypoechoic areas due to necrosis
  (ii) hyperechoic areas due to calcification or fat.
- Where renal cell carcinoma is suspected, ultrasound may also be used to look for:
  (i)   invasion of renal vein or IVC;
  (ii) lymphadenopathy;
  (iii) metastases in the liver;
  (iv) contralateral tumour.
- Ultrasound may also be used as a guide for the following procedures:
  (i)   biopsy of solid masses or complicated cysts;
  (ii) aspiration of cysts;
  (iii) cyst ablation by injection of ethanol.

2. CT

- Further characterisation of a solid mass.
- May show areas of necrosis, calcification, or fat.
- In renal cell carcinoma, CT is used to assess:
  (i)   spread into perinephric fat and invasion of local structures such as the psoas muscle;
  (ii) venous invasion;
  (iii) lymphadenopathy;
  (iv) liver metastases;
  (v)   lung metastases;
  (vi) contralateral tumour (*Fig. 16.2*).

3. MRI

- Gives similar information to CT.
- Potential advantages are:
  (i)   accurate assessment for venous invasion without the use of intravenous contrast;
  (ii) coronal plane allows accurate assessment of upper and lower renal poles.

4. Angiography

- Rarely used for renal cell carcinoma for the following:
  (i)   prior to embolisation;
  (ii) to provide a surgical 'roadmap';
  (iii) where results of cross-sectional tech-

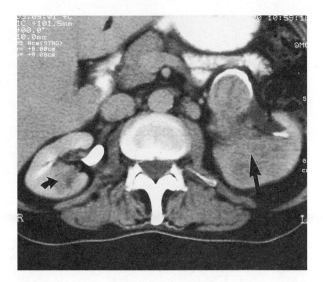

Fig. 16.2   Renal cell carcinoma – CT
Note: • irregular mass arising from the left kidney (straight arrow)
      • small contralateral tumour in the right kidney (curved arrow).

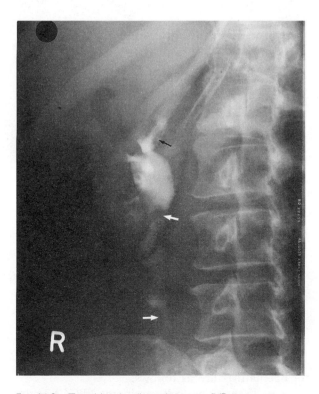

Fig. 16.3   Transitional cell carcinoma – IVP
There are numerous tumour deposits seen as irregular filling defects in the collecting system and ureter (arrows).

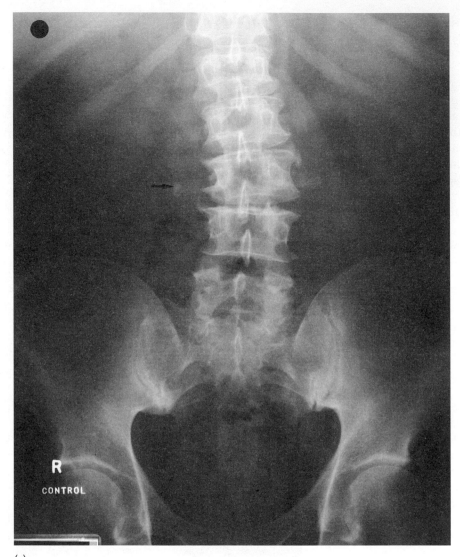

(a)

Fig. 16.4   Renal calculus
a) Plain film
Note:
• stones in both kidneys
• calculus seen projected over the tip of the right transverse process of L3 (arrow).

niques (CT and ultrasound) are equivocal with respect to venous invasion.

B. PAINLESS HAEMATURIA

In considering the investigation of haematuria one must consider the more common causes and ways to best demonstrate them. Common causes of haematuria are as follows:

• Transitional cell carcinoma (TCC) of the renal collecting system, ureter, or bladder.

• Renal cell carcinoma.
• Renal conditions such as pyelonephritis, glomerulonephritis, papillary necrosis.

I.   IVP plus cystoscopy

• IVP in combination with cystoscopy remains the best initial screening test for assessment of painless haematuria.
• IVP provides good visualisation of the calyces, renal pelvis, and ureter with anatomical detail not possible with the other modalities, e.g. a small TCC of the

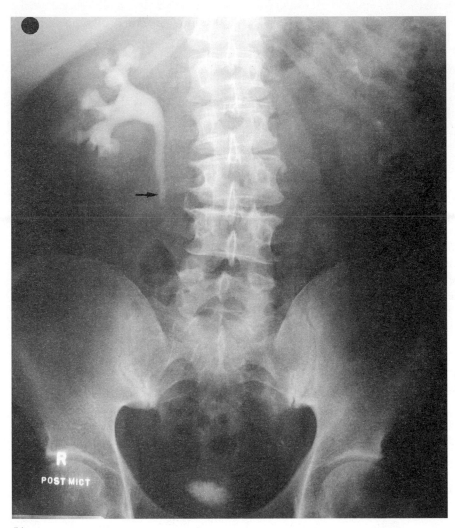

(b)

Fig. 16.4 Renal calculus
b) IVP
Note:
• dilatation of the right collecting system with 'hold-up' of contrast; compare with the normal left side
• right ureter dilated down to the level of the calculus at L3 (arrow).

renal pelvis will not be seen on CT or ultrasound unless the collecting system is dilated.

• Cystoscopy is required as IVP has relatively low accuracy in delineating the bladder.

• Signs of TCC on IVP are as follows:
  (i)   lucent filling defect;
  (ii) dilatation of the urinary tract above the tumour;
  (iii) TCCs are often multiple, so the whole urinary tract must be examined closely (*Fig. 16.3*).

• Differential diagnosis of a lucent filling defect on IVP includes: TCC, blood clot, sloughed papilla in papillary necrosis, uric acid or xanthine calculus.

• Fine-section CT is sometimes useful to further delineate a lucent filling defect: all stones will be of high attenuation on CT, even stones that are lucent on IVP and plain films.

• If a TCC or renal cell carcinoma is found, further imaging by CT and ultrasound will be required for tumour staging (see Chapter 22).

- A renal mass will be assessed as above, i.e. ultrasound initially to exclude simple cyst followed by CT if required.
- Other conditions may also be seen on IVP (e.g. pyelonephritis, papillary necrosis, etc.).

2. Ultrasound

- Ultrasound is required in the following situations:
  (i) to assess a renal mass found on IVP;
  (ii) if IVP and cystoscopy are negative, ultrasound of the kidneys should be performed; ultrasound is more sensitive than IVP for small renal masses lying outside the collecting system.
- If all imaging is negative, renal biopsy may be performed to exclude glomerulonephritis, etc.

C. RENAL COLIC

As for painless haematuria, one must consider the common causes of renal colic or renal angle pain and the best methods to demonstrate them:

- Ureteric calculus.
- Renal calculus.
- Pelvi-ureteric junction obstruction.
- Acute pyelonephritis.
- Ureteric stricture.
- TCC of the ureter causing obstruction.
- TCC of the bladder impinging on the vesico-ureteric junction.
- Clot colic, i.e. colic due to a blood clot complicating haematuria.

I. Plain films

- 90% of renal calculi contain sufficient calcium to be radio-opaque, i.e. visible on plain films.
- Cystine stones (3%) are faintly opaque.
- Urate stones (5%) are lucent.
- Xanthine and matrix stones are rare and lucent.

Note that opacities seen on plain films thought to be renal or ureteric calculi need to be differentiated from other causes of calcification (e.g. arterial calcification, calcified lymph nodes, pelvic phleboliths).

2. IVP

- Following plain films, IVP is the imaging modality of choice in the assessment of renal colic:
  (i) to prove that an opacity seen on plain films lies within the urinary tract (*Fig. 16.4*);
  (ii) to diagnose lucent calculi not seen on plain films;
  (iii) to identify other causes of renal colic, as above, and guide further actions.
- Dilatation of the entire length of the ureter with no apparent obstructing opacity is most commonly due to oedema of the vesico-ureteric junction secondary to recent passage of a calculus.
- An obstructing ureteric calculus shows all or some of the following signs:
  (i) delayed uptake of contrast by the involved kidney;
  (ii) persistent contrast outlining the renal cortex (i.e. delayed nephrogram);
  (iii) delayed appearance of contrast in the collecting system;
  (iv) dilated collecting system above the calculus;
  (v) leakage of contrast with severe obstruction;
  (vi) increased pain following injection of contrast.
- Renal calculi may be amenable to extracorporeal shock wave lithotripsy (ESWL) which uses high-focused, high-intensity ultrasound to shatter calculi into small fragments able to be passed or removed percutaneously.
- Acute pyelonephritis may show no changes on IVP or a focal deformity in the event of inflammatory mass or abscess formation.
- Pelvi-ureteric junction obstruction shows dilataton of the collecting system with marked dilatation of the renal pelvis and failure to opacify the ureter.
- Percutaneous nephrostomy may be required to salvage renal function prior to surgery.

D. RENAL TRAUMA

Imaging in renal trauma is performed for two purposes: (a) to delineate the nature of renal injuries; and (b) to detect pre-existing abnormalities, seen in up to 50% of traumatised kidneys.

1. CT with contrast (*Fig. 16.5*)

- Initial investigation of choice as it provides anatomical as well as functional information.
- Good definition of renal lacerations, haematoma, urinoma.
- Non-functioning kidney due to:
  (i) massive parenchymal damage;
  (ii) vascular pedicle injury;
  (iii) obstructed collecting system.
- CT also provides assessment of adjacent organs (e.g. liver, spleen, pancreas).

2. Ultrasound

- Provides good anatomical information with respect to renal lacerations, haematoma, urinoma.
- Adjacent organs also assessed.
- No information on renal function.

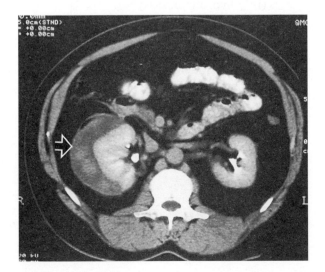

Fig. 16.5   Renal trauma – CT
Note: • normal left kidney
      • enhancing right kidney surrounded by lower attenuation perinephric haematoma (arrow).

3. IVP

- A limited IVP may be used to complement ultrasound where CT is unavailable.
- Lacerations:
  (i) well-defined defect in kidney;
  (ii) leakage of contrast.
- Intrarenal haematoma: localised filling defect with displacement of calyces.
- Differential diagnosis of non-functioning kidney, as above.
- Limitations:
  (i) imprecise information on perirenal tissues;
  (ii) adjacent organs not assessed.

4. Plain films

- Though not useful in the precise delineation of renal injuries, the following signs should alert one to the possibility of underlying renal trauma:
  (a) Loss of fat planes around the kidney and psoas margin.
  (b) Fractures of the lower 3 ribs.
  (c) Fractures of the lumbar transverse processes.
  (d) Overlying dilated loops of bowel.
  (e) Pleural effusions.

E. TRAUMA TO THE BLADDER AND URETHRA

Trauma to the bladder and/or urethra is commonly associated with pelvic fractures.

1. Plain films

- Fracture/dislocation of the pelvis (*Fig. 16.6*).
- Soft-tissue mass in the pelvis due to leakage of urine or dilatation of the bladder with acute retention.
- Air may be seen in the bladder following penetrating injury.

2. Urethrogram (*Fig. 16.7*)

- Must be performed in any patient with an anterior fracture/dislocation of the pelvis

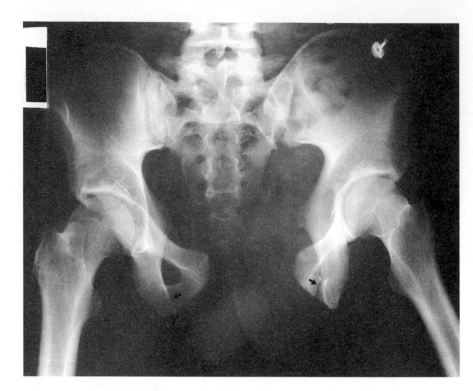

Fig. 16.6   Pelvic trauma
Note:
- separation of the pubic symphysis
- widening of the left sacro-iliac joint
- fractures of the inferior ischiopubic rami (arrows)
- soft tissue mass on the left due to haematoma.

Injuries such as this have a high incidence of associated urinary tract damage.

or with blood at the urethral meatus following trauma prior to attempted catheterisation of the bladder.

- Urethral trauma shows as:
  - (i) leakage of contrast into surrounding soft tissue planes;
  - (ii) areas of urethral irregularity or narrowing;
  - (iii) transection of the urethra with non-filling of its more proximal posterior aspect.

3.   Cystogram

- If the urethra is normal on urethrogram, a catheter can be passed into the bladder and a cystogram performed.
- If there is significant urethral damage, a suprapubic catheter should be inserted.
- Signs of bladder damge on cystogram:
  - (i) leakage of contrast: may be intraperitoneal, intrapelvic, or extrapelvic, e.g. into the soft tissue planes of the thigh;
  - (ii) distortion or displacement of the bladder due to haematoma/leakage of urine.

F.   PROSTATISM

1.   Ultrasound

- Assess kidneys for:
  - (i)   hydronephrosis;
  - (ii) calculi;
  - (iii) asymptomatic congenital anomalies and tumours.
- Assess bladder for:
  - (i)   wall thickening;
  - (ii) trabeculation and diverticulae;
  - (iii) calculi.
- Measure bladder volume pre-micturition and residual volume post-micturition – calculate by the formula: height $\times$ width $\times$ length $\times$ 0.5.
- Measure prostate volume.

2.   Plain films

- To detect renal calculi which may not be seen on ultrasound.

IVP is no longer recommended for routine use in prostatism.

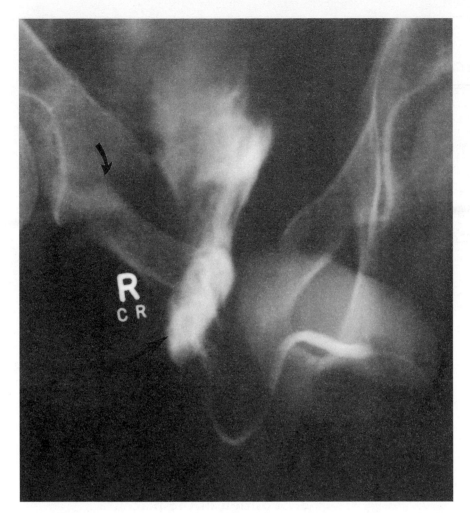

Fig. 16.7 Ruptured urethra
– urethrogram
Note:
- contrast leaking from posterior urethra (straight arrow)
- anterior pelvic fractures (curved arrow).

Further Reading

1. Amis ES, Jr (ed). Contemporary uroradiology. *Radiological Clinics in North America* 1991;**29**:3.
2. Banner MP. Interventional radiology in the urinary tract. *Current Imaging* 1989;**1**:10–20.
3. Evans C. The intravenous urogram. *Current Imaging* 1989;**1**:114–118.
4. Fidas A, Mackinlay JY, Wild SR, Chisholm GD. Ultrasound as an alternative to intravenous urography in prostatism. *Clinical Radiology* 1987;**38**:479–482.
5. Fry IK, Cattell WR. The nephrographic pattern during excretory urography. *British Medical Bulletin* 1972;**28**:227–231.
6. Kelly IMG, Lees WR, Rickards D. Prostate cancer and the role of color Doppler US. *Radiology* 1993;**189**: 153–156.
7. Pollack HM, Resnick MI. Prostate-specific antigen and screening for prostate cancer: much ado about something. *Radiology* 1993;**189**:353–356.
8. Slonim SM, Cuttino JT, Johnson CJ et al. Diagnosis of prostatic carcinoma: value of random transrectal sonographically guided biopsies. *AJR* 1993;**161**: 1003–1006.

17
Female reproductive system

A. The 'routine' obstetrical scan
B. Ultrasound in gynaecology
C. Investigation of a breast lump
D. Investigation of nipple discharge
E. Breast screening

A. THE 'ROUTINE' OBSTETRICAL SCAN

The word 'routine' appears in inverted commas because there really is no such thing as a routine obstetrical scan. I say this despite the fact that in Western society the majority of pregnant women will have an ultrasound scan. The obstetrical scan should only be performed when the referring doctor and patient have a clear view of the benefits and limitations of the technique. The potential implications of an abnormal finding should be understood prior to the examination. Having said that, the best time for such a scan is at 18–20 weeks' gestation. This provides accurate dating, as well as a good assessment of foetal morphology.

The findings of obstetrical ultrasound scans are as follows.

1. Number of foetuses

2. Assessment of gestational age

- Measurements of biparietal diameter and femur length (*Fig. 17.1*).
- Accurate to ± 1 week

3. Position of the placenta

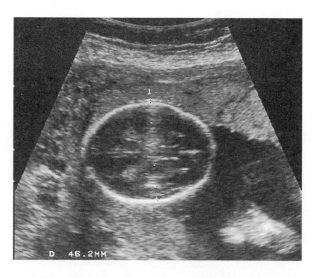

Fig. 17.1 Biparietal diameter measurement – ultrasound.

4. Liquor volume

5. Foetal morphology

- *Head*:
  - outline of skull bones;
  - cerebral ventricles;
  - posterior fossa;
  - falx cerebri;
  - facial sections for cleft palate.
- *Spine*:
  - ossification centres;
  - overlying skin line;
  - nuchal fold thickness (may be increased in Down's syndrome).
- *Thorax*:
  - cardiac activity;
  - four-chamber view of heart;
  - aortic arch;
  - diaphragm.
- *Abdomen*:
  - stomach (filled with fluid);
  - kidneys;
  - bladder;
  - umbilical cord insertion (exclude omphalocele);
  - ensure 3 vessels in cord (2 vessels associated with foetal anomalies).
- *Extremities*:
  - arms/legs;
  - hands/feet.

6. Detection of maternal pelvic masses or cysts

Note that obstetrical scans may be performed earlier in pregnancy for a variety of reasons:

- First trimester bleeding/pain – up to 12 weeks' gestation transvaginal ultrasound may be used.
- Clinical suspicion of an abnormality:
  (i) large for dates;
  (ii) abnormal alpha-foetoprotein.

Scans may also be required later in pregnancy for a variety of reasons:

- Follow up of placenta praevia – the majority of placenta praevia diagnosed on the 18–20 weeks' scan will resolve later in pregnancy with increased growth of the lower uterine segment producing apparent upward 'migration' of the placenta.
- Follow-up of foetal abnormality.
- Suspected growth retardation.
- Maternal problems (e.g. diabetes).
- Guidance of amniocentesis or other interventions.

B. ULTRASOUND IN GYNAECOLOGY

Ultrasound is the primary investigation of choice for assessment of pelvic masses. Masses are characterised by ultrasound as cystic, solid, or mixed. Organ of origin (i.e. uterus, ovary, other pelvic organs) may be ascertained. Ultrasound is used in a wide variety of clinical situations (e.g. suspected ectopic pregnancy, assessment of endometriosis, infertility).

Two types of ultrasound examinations are available:

I. Transabdominal

- Requires a full bladder to push small bowel loops out of the way and so provide an 'acoustic window' to the pelvic organs.
- Good for larger masses or cysts.
- May also assess complications such as hydronephrosis, ascites, liver metastases.

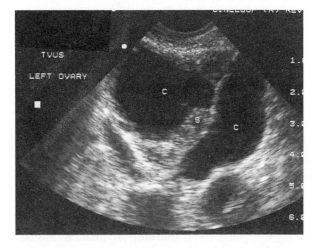

Fig. 17.2 Cystadenocarcinoma of the ovary – transvaginal ultrasound.
Note cystic components (c), separated by a thick soft tissue septum (s).

2. Transvaginal (*Fig. 17.2*)

- Empty bladder required.
- Higher-frequency probes are used giving better anatomical resolution of the uterus and ovaries.
- Major limitation is smaller field of view, so unable to fully assess large pelvic masses or kidneys for complications such as hydronephrosis.
- May be inappropriate for very young or elderly patients.
- Apart from these constraints, the transvaginal technique is more accurate than transabdominal scanning in early pregnancy (up to 12 weeks' gestation) and in most gynaecological conditions.
- Transvaginal ultrasound may be used to guide interventional procedures (e.g. biopsy, cyst aspiration, abscess drainage, ovarian harvest, etc.) in IVF programmes

Classification of pelvic masses based on ultrasound appearances and organ of origin is as follows:

(a) Cysts:

- Simple ovarian cyst.
- Hydrosalpinx.
- Endometrioma.

(b) Solid masses:

(i) Uterus
  - Fibroid.
  - Uterine sarcoma/carcinoma.
(ii) Ovary
  - Fibroma.
  - Brenner tumour.

(c) Mixed lesions

Mixed lesions, i.e. cysts with internal echoes or solid components such as soft tissue septae, wall thickening, or associated soft tissue mass:
(i) Uterus
  - Degenerate fibroid.
  - Necrosis in uterine sarcoma/carcinoma.
(ii) Ovary/Fallopian tube
  - Ectopic pregnancy.
  - Ovarian tumour: dermoid cyst; serous/mucinous tumour.

- Endometrioma.
- Pelvic inflammatory disease.

For further notes on staging of gynaecological tumours see Chapter 22.

C. INVESTIGATION OF A BREAST LUMP

1. Mammography

- Mammography is useful in the characterisation of a palpable breast mass.
- Features of a benign mass:
  (a) well-defined margin;
  (b) surrounding lucent halo;
  (c) homogeneous density;

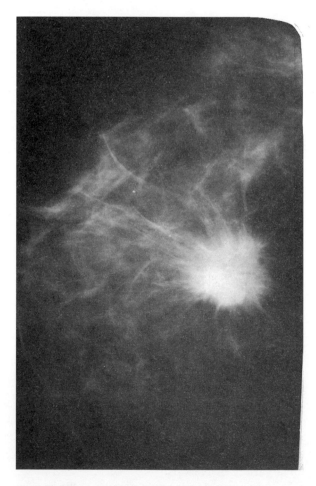

Fig. 17.3 Breast carcinoma – mammogram
Note the features of a malignant mass:
- irregular margin
- high density.

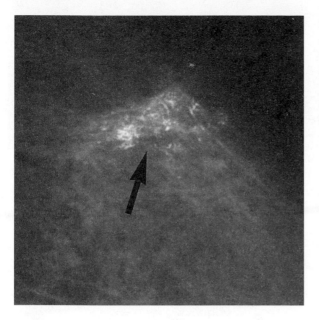

Fig. 17.4 Malignant microcalcification – mammogram Dense cluster of irregular, branching-type calcification (arrow).

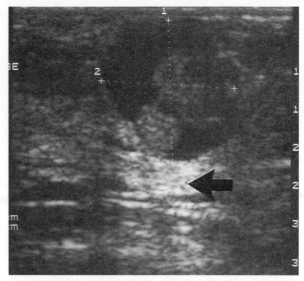

Fig. 17.5 Complicated cyst – ultrasound
Note:
- well-defined hypoechoic structure
- acoustic enhancement (arrow)
- two soft tissue structures within the anechoic fluid; these were papillomas growing in an otherwise simple cyst.

(d) low or medium density, i.e. normal structures like blood vessels can be seen through the mass;
(e) benign calcification.
- Features of a malignant mass (*Fig. 17.3*):
  (a) ill-defined irregular margin;
  (b) non-homogeneous density;
  (c) high density, i.e. normal structures cannot be seen through the mass;
  (d) malignant-type calcification (*Fig. 17.4*);
  (e) secondary signs: nipple retraction, skin thickening, distortion of surrounding architecture.

2. Ultrasound (*Fig. 17.5*)

- In the absence of calcification benign masses and cysts are often difficult to distinguish from each other on mammography.
- The traditional role for ultrasound in breast disease has been differentiation of simple cysts from solid lesions.
- As for other parts of the body, the criteria of a simple cyst are:

(a) anechoic contents;
(b) well-defined thin wall;
(c) acoustic enhancement.
- Should these criteria not be met further assessment is needed (e.g. cyst aspiration, biopsy, surgical removal).
- Ultrasound is also useful in the characterisation of masses poorly seen on mammography due to density of the surrounding breast stroma: this is particularly so in younger women who tend to have quite dense breasts on mammography.

D. INVESTIGATION OF NIPPLE DISCHARGE

1. Mammography

- Underlying mass or calcification.

2. Galactography

- May be used if the discharge is unilateral from a single duct: a higher positive rate is seen with blood-stained discharge.

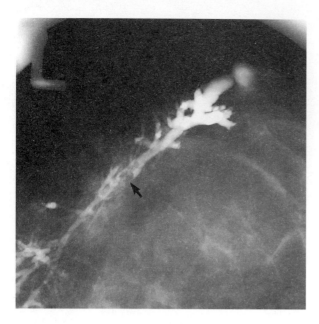

Fig. 17.6   Intraduct papilloma – galactogram
Note: • contrast filled duct system
       • papilloma shows as an irregular filling defect
         (arrow).

- The duct orifice is gently cannulated with a fine catheter and a small amount of contrast injected.
- Intraduct papilloma: smooth or irregular filling defect in the contrast-filled duct (*Fig. 17.6*).
- Invasive carcinoma: irregular narrowing of the duct with distal dilatation.
- Duct ectasia: generalised dilatation of the main duct and its branches.

E. BREAST SCREENING

- Mammographic screening for breast cancer is of benefit in reducing mortality in the over-50 age group.
- There is as yet no proven benefit for women below this age.

- The aims of a screening programme are early detection of cancers and a reduction in mortality in the 55–69 age group.
- A dedicated team is essential comprising radiographer, radiologist, surgeon, pathologist, and counselling nurse.
- Strict quality control over equipment, film processing, and training of personnel is essential.
- An abnormality found on initial screening mammogram (e.g. mass, suspicious microcalcification) leads to recall of the patient and a second stage of investigation:
  (i)   clinical assessment;
  (ii) ultrasound;
  (iii) further mammographic views of the suspicious area including magnification views;
  (iv) fine-needle aspiration of palpable lesions;
  (v)   radiological localisation and biopsy of non-palpable lesions.
- If after this second stage a lesion is found to be malignant, the patient is referred for surgery; if benign, she is brought back for routine screening; indeterminate lesions would usually undergo open biopsy or be reassessed after 1 year.

Further Reading

1. Gordon PB, Goldenberg SL, Chan NHL. Solid breast lesions: diagnosis with US-guided fine-needle aspiration biopsy. *Radiology* 1993;**189**:573–580.
2. Guyer PB. The role of ultrasound in breast disease. *Current Imaging* 1989;**1**:100–107.
3. Mendelson EB, Bohm-velez M, Neiman HL, Russo J. Transvaginal sonography in gynaecologic imaging. *Seminars in Ultrasound, CT and MR* 1988;**9**:102–121.
4. O'Brien GD, Robinson HP, Warren P. The 18 to 20 week obstetrical scan. *MJA* 1993;**158**:567–570.
5. Tabar L, Dean PB. *Teaching Atlas of Mammography*, 2nd edn. Thieme, 1985.

18
Skeletal system

A. Anatomy of a growing bone
B. Subtle fractures
C. Complications of fractures
D. Approach to arthropathies
E. Osteoporosis
F. Imaging of joints

In this chapter, I have attempted to focus on selected problem areas to do with bones and joints. I have not attempted a comprehensive review of orthopaedics, for such an exercise would double the size of this book! Excellent classifications of fractures and their radiographic appearances are available in a wide range of books. My personal favourite is *Apley's System of Orthopaedics and Fractures.* I shall therefore deal with the following topics:

- Anatomy of growing bone.
- Subtle fractures.
- Complications of fractures.
- Approach to arthropathies.
- Assessment of osteoporosis.
- Imaging of joints.

The spine is considered in a separate chapter, as are skull and facial fractures; for notes on arthrography see Chapter 7.

A. ANATOMY OF A GROWING BONE (*Fig. 18.1*)

Bones develop and grow through primary and secondary ossification centres. Virtually all primary centres are present at birth. The part of

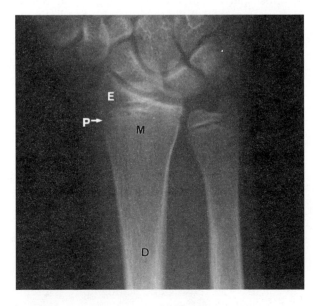

Fig. 18.1 Anatomy of a growing bone
Note: • epiphysis (E)
     • epiphyseal cartilage or growth plate (P)
     • metaphysis (M)
     • diaphysis (D).

bone ossified from the primary centre is termed the *diaphysis*. In long bones the diaphysis forms most of the shaft. Secondary ossification centres occur later in growing bones, most appearing after birth. The secondary centre at the end of a growing long bone is termed the *epiphysis*. The epiphysis is separated from the shaft of the bone by the epiphyseal growth cartilage or *physis*. An *apophysis* is another type of secondary ossification centre which forms a protrusion from the growing bone. Examples of apophyses include the greater trochanter of the femur and the tibial tuberosity. The *metaphysis* is that part of the bone between the diaphysis and the physis. The diaphysis and metaphysis are covered by periosteum, and the articular surface of the epiphysis is covered by articular cartilage.

B. SUBTLE FRACTURES

Obvious fractures are just that – obvious, and can often be diagnosed by the patient holding the X-ray up to the ceiling light! The diagnosis of fractures that display subtle X-ray changes is important and often difficult. There is no substitute for careful history and examination followed by close perusal of the tender region on X-ray. Fractures can be difficult to see for a number of reasons, as below.

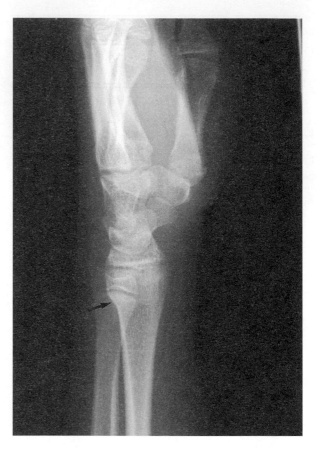

Fig. 18.2 Buckle (torus) fracture
There is a buckle in the posterior cortex of the distal radius without a definite cortical break (arrow).

1.   Minimal displacement

- Often referred to as 'hairline' fractures.
- Oblique fractures of the long bones can be especially difficult, particularly in paediatric patients.
- Fractures through the waist of the scaphoid can also be difficult in the acute phase; owing to the risk of avascular necrosis of the proximal pole of the scaphoid, it is recommended that regardless of the initial X-ray result, all patients with clinically suspected scaphoid fracture be treated and have a repeat X-ray in 7–10 days; bone scintigraphy is useful in doubtful cases.

2.   Paediatric fractures

- Children tend to have softer, more malleable bones which may not completely fracture.
- Buckle (torus) fracture: bend in the cortex without actual cortical break; common in the distal radius (*Fig.18.2*).
- Green stick fracture: only one cortex is broken with bending of the other cortex (*Fig.18.3*).
- Fractures in and around the epiphysis may be difficult to see and are classified by the Salter Harris system, as follows:
  (i)   Salter Harris 1: epiphyseal plate (i.e. cartilage) fracture (*Fig. 18.4*).
  (ii) Salter Harris 2: fracture of metaphysis with/without displacement of epiphysis.
  (iii) Salter Harris 3: fracture of epiphysis only.

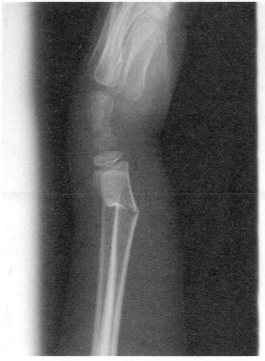

Fig. 18.3 Greenstick fracture
Note: • buckling of posterior cortex
• break in anterior cortex.

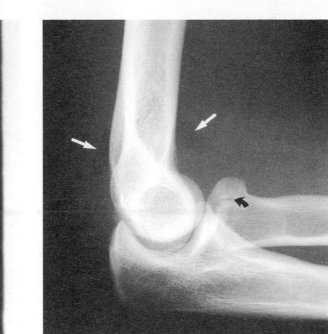

Fig. 18.5 Elbow joint effusion
Note: • elevation of the anterior fat pad and posterior
fat pads (straight arrows)
• fracture of the radial head (curved arrow).

(iv) Salter Harris 4: fracture of both meta-physis and epiphysis.
(v) Salter Harris 5: impaction and compression of the epiphyseal plate.
• Types 1 and 5 are the most difficult to appreciate as the bones themselves are intact: they are important to diagnose, however, as untreated disruption of the epiphyseal plate may lead to problems with growth of the bone.

3. Fractures in complex areas

• These fractures are difficult to diagnose radiographically due to overlapping structures.
• Examples include: the pelvis, especially the acetabulum; the feet, particularly the tarsal bones; the wrist, particularly less common fractures such as fracture of the hook of hamate.
• Strategies for diagnosis of suspected fractures in these regions include:

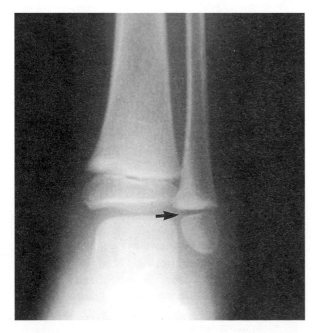

Fig. 18.4 Salter-Harris Type 1 fracture
There is angulation of the distal epiphysis of the fibula
with widening of the epiphyseal plate medially (arrow).

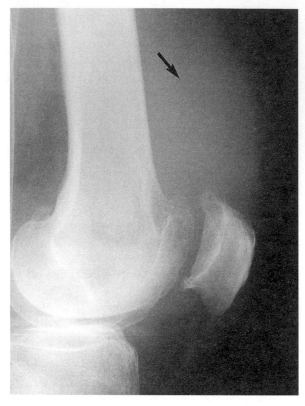

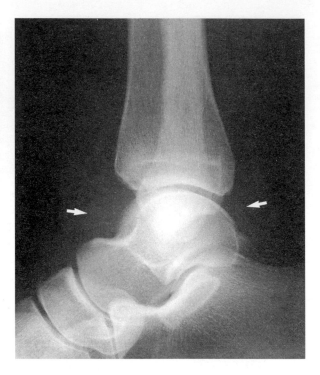

Fig. 18.7   Ankle joint effusion
The ankle joint is distended anteriorly and posteriorly by fluid (arrows).

Fig. 18.6   Knee joint effusion
Note the appearance of a large, soft tissue mass above the patella. This is due to fluid filling and distending the suprapatellar pouch of the knee joint (arrow).

(i)   further radiographic views: obliques, stress views;

(ii)   recognition of joint effusions – effusions are easily recognised in the elbow, knee, and ankle joints (*Figs. 18.5, 18.6,* and *18.7*); the finding of a fluid-fluid level in the knee joint due to lipo-haemarthrosis is particularly suggestive of a fracture often of the tibial plateau seen on oblique views (*Fig. 18.8*).

(iii)   scintigraphy – ^{99m}Tc-MDP; will be positive within 24 hours of a fracture;

(iv)   CT – fine sections through the area of interest (*Fig. 18.9*); particularly good for giving further anatomical detail prior to surgery; this function is especially applicable to comminuted fractures of the calcaneus and also of the acetabulum where 3D reconstruction may also be used.

4.   Stress fractures

- A stress fracture is a fracture occurring in a normal bone due to prolonged, repetitive muscle action on that bone.
- Stress fractures are particularly common in people engaged in sports, ballet, and gymnastics and a wide range of stress fractures has been described occurring in particular activities.
- X-rays are often normal at the time of initial presentation.
- After 7–10 days, periosteal thickening is usually visible, as well as a faint fracture line.
- Scintigraphy:
  (i) ^{99m}Tc-MDP;
  (ii)   usually positive at the time of initial presentation.

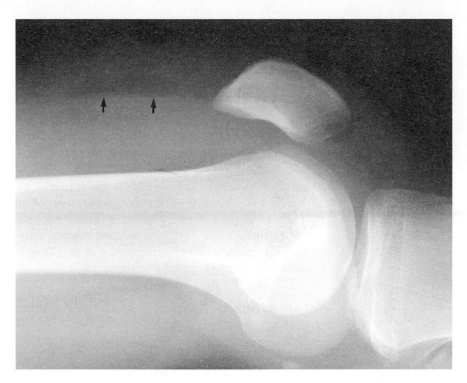

Fig. 18.8 Knee joint lipo-haemarthrosis
Note low-density fat floating on higher-density blood in the suprapatellar pouch of the knee joint. This produces a fluid–fluid level (arrows) and indicates release of fat into the knee joint from a fracture. In this case, there was a fracture of the upper tibia.

- CT: useful for stress fractures in complex areas difficult to see with conventional X-rays (e.g. the talar dome or navicular in runners).

C. COMPLICATIONS OF FRACTURES

1. Delayed union

- Occurs due to incomplete immobilisation, infection at the fracture site, pathological fractures, i.e. fractures through an underlying bone lesion, vitamin C deficiency, or in elderly patients.

2. Mal-union

- Union has occurred, though in a poor position leading to bone or joint deformity and often to early osteoarthritis.

3. Non-union

- This term implies that the bone will never unite without some form of intervention.

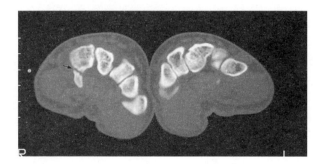

Fig. 18.9 Fracture of the hook of hamate – CT
A fracture line through the base of the hook of the hamate is elegantly demonstrated with CT (arrow).

- Two appearances may be seen:
  (i) sclerosis (i.e. increased density) of the bone ends with a lucent margin between them;
  (ii) fracture line able to be seen through surrounding callus.

4. Avascular necrosis (*Fig. 18.10*)

- Occurs most commonly in 3 sites: proximal pole of scaphoid, femoral head, body of talus.

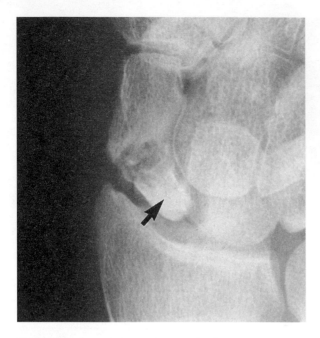

Fig. 18.10   Avascular necrosis complicating scaphoid fracture
Note: • non-union of a fracture through the waist of the scaphoid
      • increased density of the proximal pole of the scaphoid indicating avascular necrosis (arrow).

- Due to interruption of blood supply as may occur in fractures of the waist of the scaphoid, femoral neck, and neck of talus.
- The non-vascularised portion of bone becomes sclerotic over 2–3 months; this is due to new bone being laid down on necrosed bone trebaculae.
- Due to weight-bearing, the femoral head and talus may show irregularity and deformity, as well as sclerosis.

5.   Sudeck's atrophy

- Sudeck's atrophy may be considered as a severe form of disuse osteoporosis which may follow major or trivial bone injury.
- Occurs in bones distal to the site of injury.
- Associated with severe pain and swelling.
- X-ray changes:
  (i)   severe decrease in bony density distal to fracture site;
  (ii) marked thinning of bony cortex;

- Scintigraphy:
  (i) ^{99m}Tc-MDP;
  (ii) increased uptake in the limb distal to the trauma site.

D.   APPROACH TO ARTHROPATHIES

Many classifications of joint diseases are available based on differing criteria (e.g. X-ray appearances, aetiology, etc.). I find it most useful to decide first whether there is involvement of a single joint (monoarthropathy) or multiple joints (polyarthropathy). This is fine as long as one remembers that a polyarthropathy may present early with a single painful joint.

(a)   Monoarthropathy

1.   Trauma

- Usually an obvious history.
- Associated fracture and joint effusion.

2.   Septic arthritis

- Joint may be radiographically normal at time of initial presentation.
- Later a joint effusion and swelling of surrounding soft tissues may occur, followed by bone erosions and destruction.
- Scintigraphy (^{99m}Tc-MDP): usually positive at time of presentation.

3.   Gout

- See following notes.

4.   Osteoarthritis

- See following notes.

5.   Early presentation of rheumatoid arthritis

- See following notes.

(b)   Polyarthropathy

1.   Inflammatory

- Painful joints with associated soft tissue swelling.

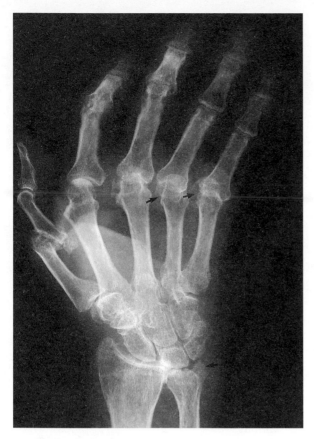

Fig. 18.11   Rheumatoid arthritis
Note: • decreased bone density
 • erosion of the metacarpophalangeal and
   proximal interphalangeal joints, and of the ulnar
   styloid (arrows)
 • subluxation of the metacarpophalangeal joints.

(A) Rheumatoid arthritis (RA) (Fig. 18.11)

- symmetrical distribution;
- affects predominantly the small joints, especially metacarpo-phalangeal, meta-tarso-phalangeal, carpal, proximal inter-phalangeal;
- soft tissue swelling overlying joints is an early sign;
- erosions:
   (i) occur earlier in the feet than the hands;
   (ii) affect metatarsal and metacarpal heads, articular surfaces of phalanges, and carpal bones;

- periarticular osteoporosis;
- abnormalities of joint alignment:
   (i) subluxation of MCP joints: ulnar deviation;
   (ii) subluxation of MTP joints: lateral deviation of toes;
- axial involvment is rare apart from the cervical spine where erosion of the odontoid peg is the most significant feature.

(B) Other connective tissue (seropositive) arthropathies:

   (i) SLE;
   (ii) systemic sclerosis;
   (iii) CREST;
   (iv) mixed connective tissue disease;
   (v) polymyositis;
   (vi) dermatomyositis.

- tend to present with symmetrical arthropathy involving the peripheral small joints, especially the metacarpo-phalangeal and proximal interphalangeal joints;
- soft tissue swelling and periarticular osteoporosis;
- erosions less common than with RA;
- soft tissue calcification, especially around joints;
- alignment deformities;
- generalised osteoporosis and avascular necrosis of the hip may complicate steroid therapy;
- resorption of distal phalanges and joint contractures are features of systemic sclerosis.

(C) Seronegative inflammatory arthropathies

   (i) ankylosing spondylitis: may occur alone or associated with ulcero-inflammatory bowel disease (i.e. Crohn's disease or ulcerative colitis);
   (ii) Reiter's syndrome;
   (iii) psoriatic arthropathy;
   (iv) juvenile chronic arthritis.

- asymmetrical polyarthropathies usually involving few joints;
- predilection for spine and sacro-iliac joints, especially ankylosing spondylitis;
- spine changes:

(i) syndesmophytes – vertically orientated bony spurs arising from the vertebral bodies;

(ii) ankylosis giving 'bamboo spine';

- sacro-iliac joints:
  (i) early erosions with an irregular joint margin;
  (ii) later sclerosis and joint fusion;
- peripheral joints:
  (i) more commonly affected with Reiter's syndrome (feet) and psoriatic arthropathy (feet and hands);
  (ii) asymmetrical distribution;
  (iii) periarticular erosions;
  (iv) periosteal new bone formation;
  (v) osteoporosis less prominent than with RA.

2. Degenerative (i.e. osteoarthritis, OA) (*Fig.18.12*)

- Primary: no underlying cause.
- Secondary: underlying arthropathy (e.g. RA), trauma, Paget's disease.

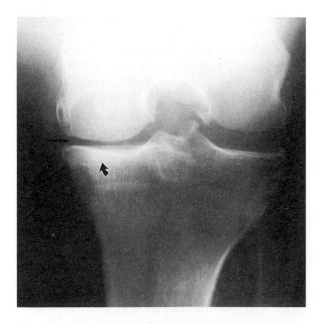

Fig. 18.12   Osteoarthritis of the knee
Note: • joint space narrowing most severe medially (straight arrow)
- osteophyte formation
- peri-articular sclerosis (curved arrow).

- Distribution of primary OA:
  (i) asymmetric;
  (ii) large weight-bearing joints: hips, knees;
  (iii) lumbar spine;
  (iv) cervical spine;
  (v) distal interphalangeal, first carpometacarpal, and lateral carpal joints.
- Joint space narrowing.
- Osteophyte formation.
- Periarticular sclerosis.
- Periarticular erosion and cyst formation.
- Loose bodies due to detached osteophytes and ossified cartilage debris.

3. Metabolic

(a) Gout
- Distribution:
  (i) first metatarso-phalangeal joint in 70%;
  (ii) other joints of lower limbs: ankles, knees, intertarsal joints;
  (iii) asymmetric, often monoarticular.

Acute gout:
- soft tissue swelling;
- no bony changes.

Chronic gouty arthritis:
- occurs with recurrent acute gout;
- erosions – para-articular on the medial and dorsal aspects around the first metatarso-phalangeal joint;
- calcification of articular cartilages, especially the menisci of the knee;
- tophi – soft tissue masses in the synovium of joints, the subcutaneous tissues of the lower leg, Achilles' tendon, olecranon bursa, helix of the ear; calcification uncommon.

(b) Amyloidosis
(c) Multicentric reticulohistiocytosis
(d) Hyperlipidaemia

E. OSTEOPOROSIS

Osteoporosis may be defined as a condition in which the quantity of bone per unit volume (i.e. bone mineral density, BMD) is decreased in amount. Osteoporosis may be generalised or localised, primary or secondary (e.g. in rheumatoid arthritis). BMD is the most important determinant of bone fragility; accurate measurement of BMD is therefore important in the early diagnosis of osteoporosis and in follow-up of therapy.

1. Dual X-ray absorptiometry (DEXA)

- Widely accepted as a highly accurate, low radiation dose technique for measuring BMD.
- Uses an X-ray source which produces X-rays of two different energies. The lower of these energies is absorbed almost exclusively by soft tissue. The higher energy is absorbed by bone and soft tissue. Calculation of the two absorption patterns gives an attenuation profile of the bone component from which BMD may be estimated.
- Measurements are usually taken from the lumbar spine (L2–L4) and the femoral neck.

2. Dual photon absorptiometry

- Uses a radionuclide source with two different energies (^{153}Gd).
- Same principles as DEXA.
- More expensive than DEXA, plus greater logistical difficulties with handling of radionuclide.

3. Quantitative CT

- Much more complex technique than DEXA.
- More expensive; higher radiation dose.

4. Quantitative ultrasound

- Not universally accepted at present.

F. IMAGING OF JOINTS

1. Wrist

Imaging methods for the wrist include:
- Plain films: stress views;
- Scintigraphy;
- CT;
- Arthrography;
- MRI.

(a) *Suspected fracture*:
- Plain films.

(b) *Scaphoid fracture*:
- Plain films – oblique views; films at 7–10 days.
- Scintigraphy in doubtful cases.

(c) *Carpal instability* (e.g. post-trauma):
- Plain films with stress views.
- Arthrography.

(d) *Triangular fibrocartilage complex injury*:
- Arthrography.
- MRI.

2. Shoulder

Imaging methods available for assessment of the shoulder are as follows:
- Plain films;
- Ultrasound;
- Arthrography;
- Arthrography with CT (*Fig. 18.13*);
- MRI (*Fig. 18.14*).

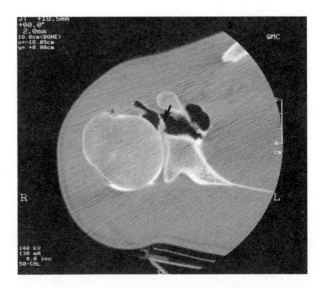

Fig. 18.13   Labral tear – CT arthrogram
Note: • the joint has been injected with air and contrast
- a mass in the anterior joint space (arrow) due to an anterior tear of the superior labrum; this is an example of a SLAP (superior labrum anterior to posterior) lesion, i.e. tear of the superior labrum at the attachment of the long head of biceps tendon.

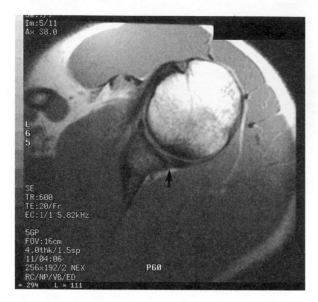

Fig. 18.14 Posterior labral tear – MRI
A high-signal line (arrow) crossing the low-signal posterior labrum indicates a tear.

(a) *Rotator cuff disease*:
 • Plain films:
   (i)   exclude underlying bony pathology;
   (ii) assess acromio-clavicular joint;
   (iii) downward-projecting osteophytes may cause impingement on the rotator cuff;
 • Ultrasound:
   (i)   very useful as initial screening test for rotator cuff tear;
   (ii) ultrasound of the rotator cuff is highly accurate when performed by radiologists experienced in the technique and using appropriate equipment;
   (iii) ultrasound is most accurate in delineating complete thickness tears, it is less sensitive for partial thickness tears.
 • Arthrography – double contrast arthrography is highly accurate for the assessment of the rotator cuff.
 • MRI:
   (i)   MRI provides excellent views of the muscles and tendons of the rotator cuff;

   (ii) its ability to image in any plane allows oblique coronal views to show the supraspinatus tendon and muscle.
(b) *Gleno-humeral instability (i.e. recurrent dislocation which may be anterior or posterior)*:
 • Plain films:
   (i)   used in initial dislocation injury;
   (ii) assess position post-reduction;
   (iii) exclude associated fractures – greater tuberosity of humerus; inferior rim of glenoid;
   (vi) exclude bony damage in recurrent dislocation – defect in postero-superior aspect of humeral head (Hill Sacks deformity); fracture of glenoid rim (Bankart lesion).
 • Arthrography with CT – CT performed immediately following double-contrast arthrography provides excellent views of the anterior and posterior cartilaginous labrum, thereafter labral tears not visible on plain films may be diagnosed.
 • MRI
(c) *Biceps tendon pathology: tendonitis/dislocation*:
 • Ultrasound – provides good visualisation of the biceps tendon and the bicipital groove.
 • CT arthrography – due to its normal communication with the shoulder joint, the biceps tendon sheath is filled with contrast and air during double-contrast arthrography.

3.   Hip

Imaging methods available are as follows:
 • Plain films;
 • CT;
 • Scintigraphy;
 • MRI;
 • Ultrasound.
(a) *Fractured neck of femur*:
 • Plain films – tomography may be helpful for undisplaced or slightly impacted femoral neck fractures.
(b) *Acetabular fractures*:
 • Plain films including oblique views.
 • CT with 3D reconstruction may assist in planning surgery.

(c) *Avascular necrosis*:
- Plain films.
- Scintigraphy.
- MRI.

(d) *Child with a limp or hip pain*:
- Plain films.
- Scintigraphy – very sensitive for early septic arthritis.
- Ultrasound – useful for diagnosis and aspiration of hip effusions, especially in very young children.

4.   Knee

Depending on local availability and practice, arthroscopy or MRI, or a combination of the two, are used in the assessment of most knee conditions (e.g. meniscus injury, cruciate ligament tear, collateral ligament tear, osteochondritis dissecans, etc.). Knee arthrography, once a common procedure, is now rarely performed where the above modalities are available.

Ultrasound is useful in the assessment of popliteal cysts and of disorders of the patellar tendon and associated bursae.

Further Reading

1.   Apley AG, Solomon L. *Apley's system of Orthopaedics and Fractures*, 7th edn. Butterworth-Heinemann, 1993.
2.   Berquist TH (ed.). *Imaging of Orthopaedic Trauma*, 2nd edn. Raven Press, 1992.
3.   Coumas JM, Waite RJ, Goss TP *et al.* CT and MR evaluation of the labral capsular ligamentous complex of the shoulder. *AJR* 1992;**158**:591–597.
4.   Daffner RH, Pavlov H. Stress fractures: current concepts. *AJR* 1992;**159**:245–252.
5.   Hunter JC, Blatz DJ, Escobedo EM. SLAP lesions of the glenoid labrum: CT arthrographic and arthroscopic correlation. *Radiology* 1992;**184**:513–518.
6.   Kaye JJ (ed.). Imaging of joints. *Radiological Clinics of North America* 1990;**28**:5.
7.   Seeger LL (ed.). *Diagnostic Imaging of the Shoulder*. Williams and Wilkins, 1992.
8.   Weiner SN, Seitz WH. Sonography of the shoulder in patients with tears of the rotator cuff: accuracy and value for selecting surgical options. *AJR* 1993;**160**:103–107.

19

Central nervous system

A. Head trauma
B. Subarachnoid haemorrhage
C. Space-occupying lesions
D. Stroke/transient ischaemic attack (TIA)

A. HEAD TRAUMA

1. Skull X-ray

For notes on the use of skull X-rays in head trauma see Chapter 6.

2. CT

- CT is the investigation of choice for the patient with significant head trauma.
- Indications:
  - (i) fractured skull with confusion, impaired consciousness, focal neurological signs or fits;
  - (ii) coma, with or without fracture;
  - (iii) deterioration in level of consciousness or development, of further neurological signs;
  - (iv) confusion or other neurological disturbance for more than 6–8 hours;
  - (v) compound depressed skull vault fracture;
  - (vi) signs of fractured base of skull, i.e. discharge of blood/CSF from ear/nose.

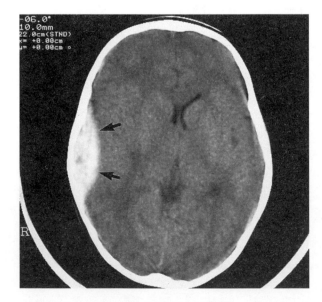

Fig. 19.1   Extradural haematoma – CT
Note: • high attenuation indicates acute haemorrhage
  • convex inner and outer margins (arrows) give the typical 'lens' shape of an extradural haematoma.

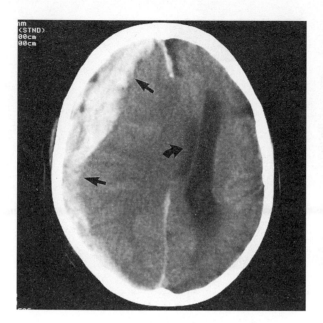

Fig. 19.2 Acute subdural haematoma – CT
Note: • high attenuation indicates acute haemorrhage
  • concave inner margin follows the surface of the brain (straight arrows)
  • marked mass effect with shift of the lateral ventricles to the left (curved arrow).

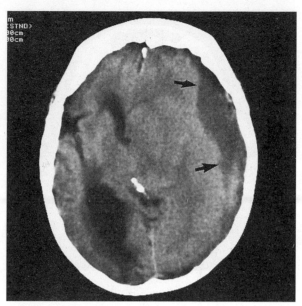

Fig. 19.3 Chronic subdural haematoma – CT
Note: • low attenuation indicates chronic haemorrhage
  • concave inner margin (arrows) indicates that the collection lies in the subdural space.

- Intracerebral haematoma:
  (i) acute intracerebral haematoma is of high attenuation (i.e. white);
  (ii) over 7–10 days the attenuation gradually decreases to approximately that of adjacent brain tissue;
  (iii) over the ensuing couple of weeks, the attenuation decreases further to approximately that of CSF (i.e. quite black).
- Extradural haematoma (*Fig. 19.1*): peripheral, high-attenuation lesion with convex inner margin.
- Subdural haematoma (*Figs. 19.2* and *19.3*):
  (i) peripheral, high-attenuation lesion with concave inner margin;
  (ii) associated swelling of underlying cerebral hemisphere contributes markedly to the associated mass effect.
- Subarachnoid haemorrhage.
- Other signs of brain damage:
  (i) contusion: mixed attenuation areas due to oedema and haemorrhage associated with mass effect (i.e. midline shift, compression of ventricles and basal cisterns);
  (ii) cerebral oedema: low-attenuation areas with associated mass effect.
- Other signs of trauma:
  (i) skull fracture: CT is especially useful in delineating base of skull fractures;
  (ii) pneumocephalus, i.e. air in the cerebral sulci or ventricles associated with fractures through sinuses or penetrating injuries;
  (iii) fluid levels in sinuses;
  (iv) foreign bodies;
  (v) scalp swelling.

3. Cervical spine

In all major trauma and head injury cases, at least a lateral cervical spine X-ray showing all 7 cervical vertebrae must be performed. For further notes see Chapter 20.

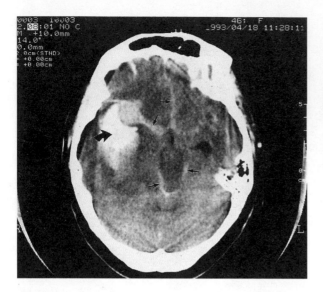

Fig. 19.4   Subarachnoid haemorrhage – CT
Subarachnoid blood is seen as high-attenuation material in the interhemispheric fissure, Sylvian fissures, and in the basal cisterns around the brain stem (straight arrows).
Note also the large intracerebral haematoma in the right temporal lobe (curved arrow).
Haemorrhage, in this case, was caused by rupture of an aneurysm of the right middle cerebral artery.

4. MRI

Owing to difficulty with visualising very acute haemorrhage, as well as relative logistical problems with monitoring equipment, etc., MRI has not displaced CT in imaging of head trauma.

B. SUBARACHNOID HAEMORRHAGE

1. CT (*Fig 19.4*)

- CT is the primary imaging investigation of choice in suspected subarachnoid haemorrhage.
- Roles of CT are as follows:
  (i) To confirm diagnosis:
- Acute subarachnoid haemorrhage shows as high-attenuation material (fresh blood) in the basal cisterns, Sylvian fissures, ventricles, and cerebral sulci.
  (ii) To suggest possible site of bleeding and/or cause:

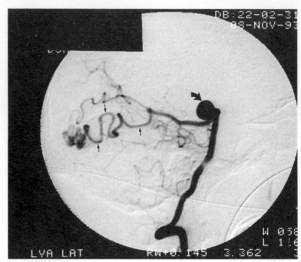

Fig. 19.5   Aneurysm and AVM – angiogram
Note: • aneurysm arising from the tip of the basilar artery (curved arrow)
  • large artery supplying a posterior AVM (straight arrows).

- By localising the greatest concentration of blood, a possible site of haemorrhage can be suggested, e.g. blood mainly in the Sylvian fissure: middle cerebral artery.
- Occasionally the cause may be seen (e.g. large aneurysm, AVM, tumour).
  (iii) To diagnose complications:
- Hydrocephalus.
- Ischaemia and infarction secondary to arterial spasm.

Note that a normal-appearing CT does not exclude subarachnoid haemorrhage. Approximately 5% of proven subarachnoid haemorrhages are missed by CT. Lumbar puncture must be performed if there is clinical suspicion of subarachnoid haemorrhage, even where the CT is negative.

2. Angiography (*Fig. 19.5*)

- Aim to show the causative lesion and direct further therapy.
- Berry aneurysm is the cause of non-traumatic subarachnoid haemorrhage in the majority (75%) of patients: angiography should show the neck of the aneurysm and exclude multiple aneurysms.

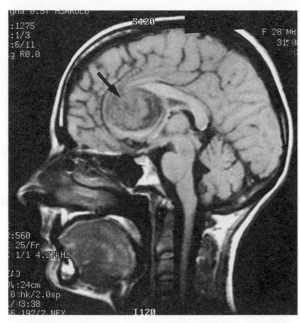

(a)

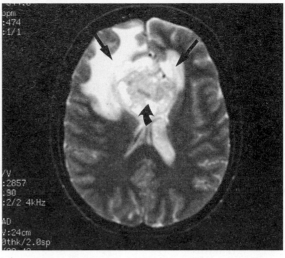

(b)

Fig. 19.6 Glioma – MRI
a) Sagittal T1-weighted scan
Note the large mass (arrow) arising from the anterior portion of the corpus callosum.
b) Axial T2-weighted scan
Note: • high-signal tumour mass (curved arrow)
        • high-signal oedema adjacent to the tumour in the frontal lobes (straight arrows).
c) Axial T1-weighted contrast scan
Enhancing tumour (arrow) can be differentiated from low-signal oedema in the frontal lobes.

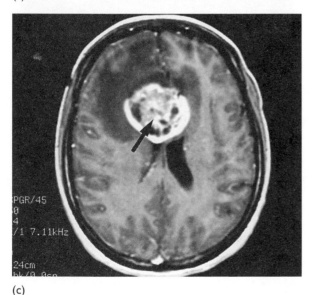

(c)

- AVM: angiography should show the anatomy of feeding arteries and draining veins; angiography may be followed by embolisation or other interventional procedures (See Chapter 8).
- Negative angiography occurs in about 15% of patients with subarachnoid haemorrhage due mainly to:
  (i) thrombosis of the aneurysm;
  (ii) vasospasm of vessels supplying the aneurysm.
- If the initial angiogram is negative, repeat angiography may be performed in 5–7 days.
- If the repeat angiogram is negative, a spinal site of bleeding should be considered and MRI of the spine performed, followed by spinal angiography for any suspicious areas.

C. SPACE OCCUPYING LESIONS

Intracranial space-occupying lesions may present clinically with:
(a) General effects (i.e. raised intracranial pressure with headaches, confusion, papilloedema).

(b) Local effects (e.g. hemiparesis, focal seizures, visual field defects).

(c) Hormonal effects in the case of functioning pituitary tumours.

The aims of imaging in suspected intracranial space-occupying lesions are as follows:

(a) Detection of a mass and differentiation from other abnormalities (e.g. hydrocephalus).

(b) Delineation of the nature of a mass.
  • Site.
  • Density; demonstration of specific contents such as calcification or fat may aid in differential diagnosis.
  • Enhancement pattern.
  • Compression or displacement of adjacent structures.

(c) Indicate and plan appropriate therapy (e.g. surgery, radiotherapy).

(d) Follow-up:
  • Assess efficacy of treatment.
  • Diagnose post-operative complications (e.g. haemorrhage, infarct).

1. MRI (*Fig. 19.6*)

  • If available, MRI would be considered the imaging investigation of choice in suspected intracranial space-occupying lesions.
  • Advantages over CT include:
    (i) better soft tissue contrast;
    (ii) multiplanar imaging;
    (iii) no image degradation due to artefact in the pituitary and posterior fossae;
    (iv) no radiation.

2. CT (*Figs. 19.7 and 19.8*)

  • Despite some limitations related to artefact in the posterior and pituitary fossae, CT remains a superb modality for assessment of suspected intracranial masses.

3. Angiography

  • Since the advent of CT and MRI, angiography is now only occasionally used for:
    (i) further characterisation of a mass (e.g. haemangioblastoma);

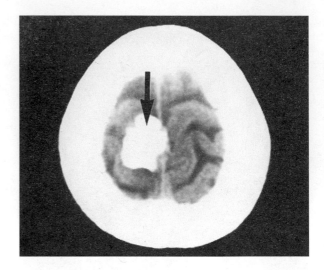

Fig. 19.7   Meningioma – CT
Densely calcified mass (arrow) arising from the falx cerebri and impinging on the supero-medial aspect of the parietal lobes.

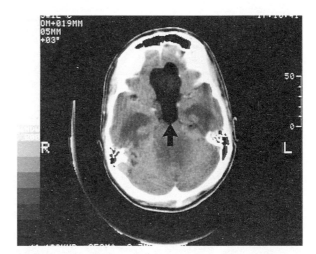

Fig. 19.8   Dermoid cyst – CT
Note: • large mass in the midline (arrow)
       • the low attenuation of the mass (less than that of CSF) indicates fat content.

    (ii) to provide a surgical 'roadmap';
    (iii) precursor to embolisation or other interventional procedures.

4.   Ultrasound

  • Though not useful in primary diagnosis, ultrasound has a minor role in localising small cerebral lesions during craniotomy when the probe can be placed directly on the brain surface.

5. Other imaging for specific situations

(a) Drop metastases, i.e. metastases via CSF to the spine seen most commonly in medulloblastoma and ependymoma.
  • MRI of the spine.
(b) Syndromes:
  • The most common example would be von Hippel-Lindau syndrome where the diagnosis of intracranial haemangioblastoma in combination with retinal angioma should lead to abdominal imaging (CT or ultrasound) to exclude an associated renal cell carcinoma.

D. STROKE/TRANSIENT ISCHAEMIC ATTACK (TIA)

I. CT (*Fig. 19.9*)

  • CT is used in the assessment of acute stroke mainly to exclude haemorrhage as the cause in patients being considered for anticoagulant therapy.
  • Whilst highly sensitive for acute haemorrhage, CT is relatively insensitive in the diagnosis of stroke of less than 24 hours' duration: changes in this time depend on the size of the stroke, and degree of associated oedema.
  • After 24 hours, infarcts show as low-attenuation areas involving grey and white matter and extending to the cerebral surface: variable degrees of mass effect may be seen with compression of ventricles and cerebral sulci.
  • As stated in the section on trauma, acute intracerebral haemorrhage shows as an area of increased attenuation.
  • Other signs of ischaemia may be seen as follows:
    (i) generalised low attenuation in the periventricular tissues;
    (ii) old infarcts – well-defined peripheral

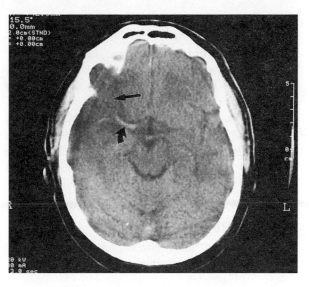

Fig. 19.9   cerebral infarct
Note: • cerebral infarct seen as a low-attenuation area in the right temporal lobe in the distribution of the right middle cerebral artery (straight arrow)
  • high attenuation in the right middle cerebral artery due to thrombosis (curved arrow).

areas of low attenuation associated with shrinkage;
    (iii) lacunar infarcts – small well-defined low-attenuation lesions in the basal ganglia and deep white matter.

2. Ultrasound (carotid duplex sonography)

  • Doppler ultrasound examination of the carotid arteries is a useful screening test able to visualise most atheromatous lesions at the carotid bifurcation.
  • Flow velocity is measured in the common carotid artery and internal carotid artery.
  • A stenosis will be indicated by:
    (i) increased flow rate;
    (ii) turbulent flow giving an abnormal Doppler wave pattern (spectral broadening).
  • Based on the above, plus the ultrasound appearance of the carotid bulb, the degree of stenosis may be quantified as follows:
    (i) up to 50%;

(ii) 50–79%;

(iii) 80–99%;

(iv) complete occlusion.

- Ultrasound has two areas of relatively poor sensitivity (though the use of colour Doppler has improved things): – ulceration of the atheromatous plaque; and occlusion of the internal carotid artery: ultrasound may miss sluggish flow in an almost occluded vessel, and as such overdiagnose complete occlusion.

3.   Angiography

- Study of the aortic arch followed by selective catheterisation of the common carotid arteries.
- Usually performed to assess stenoses of greater than 50% diameter reduction as assessed by ultrasound.
- Greater sensitivity than ultrasound for the detection of: ulceration of atheromatous plaque; and almost complete versus complete occlusion of the internal carotid artery.

4.   MRI

- MRI has greater sensitivity than CT in the assessment of stroke/TIA, in that it shows more ischaemic changes and it is more sensitive in acute lesions.
- MR angiography (MRA) shows good detail of the carotid arteries.
- With increased availability, MRI of the head with MRA of the carotid arteries may largely replace other imaging tests in the assessment of the stroke patient.

5.   Other imaging

- In a stroke/TIA patient with normal carotid arteries a search for another site of embolus may be undertaken, typically a chest X-ray and an echocardiogram.

Further Reading

1.   Archer BD. Computed tomography before lumbar puncture in acute meningitis: a review of the risks and benefits. *Can. Med. Assoc. J.* 1993;**148**:961–964.

2.   Bradley WG. MR appearance of hemorrhage in the brain. *Radiology* 1993;**189**:15–26.

3.   Bryan RN, Levy LM, Whitlow WD. Diagnosis of acute cerebral infarction of CT and MR imaging. *AJNR* 1991;**12**:611–620.

4.   Kanal E, Shellock FG. MR imaging of patients with intracranial aneursym clips. *Radiology* 1993;**187**:612–614.

5.   Lee SH, Rao KCVG, Zimmerman RA. *Cranial MRI and CT*, 3rd edn. McGraw-Hill, 1992.

20

Investigation of spine disorders

A. Spinal trauma
B. Assessment of back pain

Due to its ability to image in multiple planes, as well as its excellent soft tissue contrast, including the ability to differentiate spinal cord and nerve roots from CSF, MRI is now the imaging technique of choice in the investigation of most spine disorders. Other investigations include plain films, CT, myelography, scintigraphy, and obstetric ultrasound in the exclusion of foetal spine disorders. Plain films are still the primary investigation for spinal trauma, and this topic will be emphasised in this chapter.

A. SPINAL TRAUMA

The roles of imaging in the assessment of spinal trauma are:
- Diagnosis of fractures/dislocations.
- Assessment of stability/instability.
- Diagnosis of damage to, or impingement on, neurological structures.
- Follow-up: (a) assessment of treatment; (b) diagnosis of long-term complications (e.g. post-traumatic syrinx or cyst formation).

1. Cervical spine

(a) Plain films

Plain-film assessment of the cervical spine should be performed in all trauma patients with neck pain or tenderness, other signs of direct neck injury, or abnormal findings on neurological examination. Cervical spine films should also be performed in all patients with severe head or facial injury or following high-velocity blunt trauma or near-drowning.

The following films should be performed:
- Lateral view with patient supine showing all 7 cervical vertebrae:
  (i) traction on the shoulders may be used;
  (ii) traction on the head must *never* be used.
- Other views should also be performed with the patient supine: AP, AP open mouth to show the odontoid peg, obliques to show the facet joints and intervertebral foramina.
- Functional views, i.e. lateral views in flexion and extension with the patient erect:

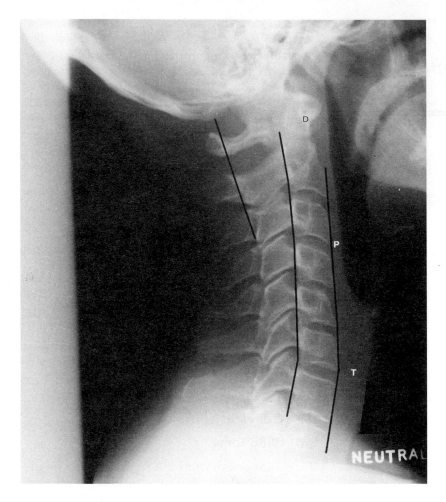

Fig. 20.1 Normal cervical spine
Note:
- anterior vertebral body line
- posterior vertebral body line
- posterior cervical line
- alignment of the facet joints
- equal spaces between spinous processes
- normal predental space (D)
- normal retropharyngeal space (P)
- normal retrotracheal space (T).

(i) performed where no fractures are seen on the neutral views to diagnose posterior or anterior ligament damage;

(ii) patient must be conscious and co-operative and must themselves perform flexion and extension, i.e. the head must not be moved passively by doctor or radiographer.

Films should be checked in a logical fashion for the following factors.

- Vertebral alignment:
  (i) disruption of anterior and posterior vertebral body lines, i.e. lines joining the anterior and posterior margins of the vertebral bodies on the lateral view;
  (ii) disruption of the posterior cervical line, i.e. a line joining the anterior aspect of the spinous processes of C1, C2, and C3; disruption of this line may indicate upper cervical spine fractures, especially of C2;
  (iii) facet joint alignment at all levels; abrupt disruption at one level may indicate locked facets;
  (iv) widening of the space between spinous processes on the lateral film;
  (v) rotation of spinous processes on the AP film;
  (vi) widening of the pre-dental space, i.e. > 5 mm in children; > 3 mm in adults.
- Bone integrity:
  (i) vertebral body fractures;
  (ii) fractures of posterior elements, i.e. pedicles, laminae, spinous processes;
  (iii) integrity of odontoid peg: anterior/ posterior/ lateral displacement.

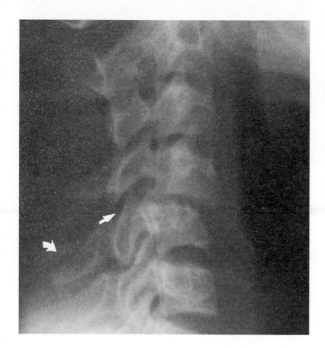

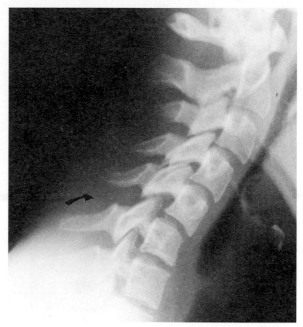

Fig. 20.2   Flexion-rotation injury at C4/C5
Note: • disruption of posterior and anterior cervical lines
       • narrowed C4/C5 disc space
       • disruption of facet joint alignment (straight arrow)
       • increased space between spinous processes of C4 and C5
       • avulsion fracture of upper surface of C5 spinous process (curved arrow).

Fig. 20.3   Soft tissue flexion injury at C5/C6
Note: • disruption of the posterior vertebral body line
       • slightly narrowed C5/C6 disc space
       • increased space between spinous processes of C5 and C6 indicates interspinous ligament damage (arrow).

• Disc spaces: narrowing or widening.
• Soft tissue changes: prevertebral swelling – widening of the retro-tracheal space, i.e. posterior aspect of trachea to C6: > 14 mm in children; > 22 mm in adults.
• Widening of the retropharyngeal space, i.e. posterior aspect of pharynx to C2: > 7 mm in adults and children (*Fig.20.1*).

Common patterns of injury are as follows.

(A) Flexion (i.e. anterior compression with posterior distraction) (Figs. 20.2 and 20.3):

• Vertebral body compression fracture.
• 'Teardrop' fracture, i.e. small triangular fragment at lower anterior margin of vertebral body.
• Disruption of posterior vertebral line.

• Disc space narrowing.
• Widening of facet joints.
• Widening of space between spinous processes.

(B) Extension (i.e. posterior compression with anterior distraction) (Figs.20.4 and 20.5):

• 'Teardrop' fracture of upper anterior margin of vertebral body: indicates severe anterior ligament damage.
• Disc space widening.
• Retrolisthesis with disruption of anterior and posterior vertebral lines.
• Fractures of posterior elements, i.e. pedicles, spinous processes, facets e.g. 'hangmans' fracture – bilateral C2 pedicle fracture.

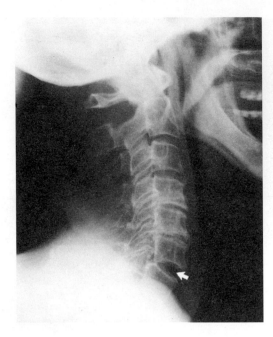

Fig. 20.4   Extension injury at C6/C7
Note: • disruption of posterior and anterior vertebral
body lines
• widening of C6/C7 disc space (arrow).

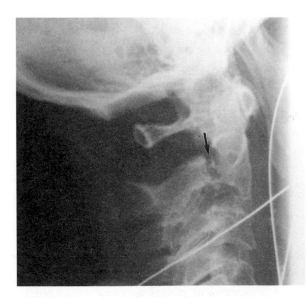

Fig. 20.5   Hangman's fracture
Note: • disruption of posterior cervical line
• fractures of the pedicles of C2 (arrow).

(C) Rotation:

- Anterolisthesis with disruption of posterior vertebral line.
- Lateral displacement of upper vertebral body on AP view.
- Abrupt disruption of alignment of facet joints: locked facets.
- Narrow disc space.
- Rotation of spinous processes on AP film.

Instability implies the possibility of increased spinal deformity or neurological damage occurring with continued stress. Signs of instability are:

- Displacement of vertebral body.
- 'Teardrop' fractures of vertebral body.
- Odontoid peg fracture.
- Widening or disruption of alignment of facet joints including locked facets.
- Widening of space between spinous processes.
- Fractures at multiple levels.

(b) CT

- Further delineation of fractures and associated deformity.
- More accurate assessment, especially of neural arches and facet joints.
- Accurate estimation of dimensions of spinal canal.

(c) MRI (*Fig. 20.6*)

- Has replaced myelography for the assessment of spinal cord damage:
  (i)   transection;
  (ii) swelling/oedema/haemorrhage;
  (iii) cyst and syrinx formation.
- Soft tissue changes:
  (i)   disc lesions;
  (ii) spinal canal haematoma.

2. Thoracic and lumbar spine

(a) Plain films

Assessment of plain films of the thoracic and lumbar spine following trauma is similar to that outlined for the cervical spine with particular attention to the following factors:

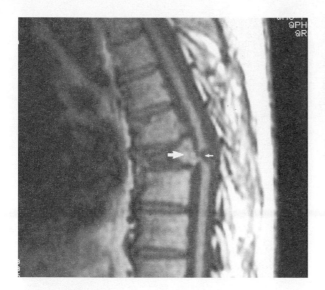

Fig. 20.6 Thoracic spine fracture – MRI
Note: • localised kyphosis due to a vertebral body crush
           fracture
       • bone fragment in the spinal canal impinging on
         the spinal cord (large arrow)
       • post-traumatic cyst formation in the spinal cord
         (small arrow).

• Vertebral alignment.
• Vertebral body height.
• Disc space height.
• Facet joint alignment.
• Space between spinous processes.
• Distance between pedicles on AP film:
  widening at one level may indicate a burst
  fracture of the vertebral body.

Common patterns of injury are:

(A) Burst fracture:

• Fractures of the vertebral body with a
  fragment pushed posteriorly into the
  spinal canal.

(B) Compression fracture:

• Loss of height of vertebral body.

(C) Fracture/dislocation:

• Vertebral body displacement.
• Disc space narrowing or widening.
• Fractures of neural arches, including facet
  joints.

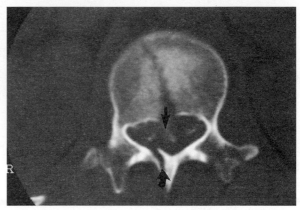

Fig. 20.7 Lumbar spine fracture – CT
Note: • fracture of the vertebral body
       • fracture of the right lamina (curved arrow)
       • bone fragments in the spinal canal (straight
         arrow).

• Widening of facet joints or space between
  spinous processes.

(D) Chance fracture (seatbelt fracture):

• Fracture of posterior vertebral body.
• Horizontal fracture line through spinous
  process, laminae, pedicles, transverse
  processes.
• Most occur at thoraco-lumbar junction.
• High association with abdominal injury
  (i.e. solid organ damage, intestinal perforation).

Signs of instability are:

• 3-column approach.
  (i) the spine may be divided into 3
      vertical columns passing respectively
      through the anterior, middle, and
      posterior thirds of the vertebral
      bodies;
  (ii) fractures of the middle and/or poste-
      rior columns are considered unstable.
• Other signs as for cervical spine, i.e. vertebral body displacement, fractures at
  multiple levels, widening of facet joints or
  spinous processes.

(b) CT (*Fig. 20.7*)

• More accurate delineation of fractures
  and deformity.

- Spinal canal well visualised in cross-section: posterior fragments impinging on spinal canal.

(c) MRI

- Assessment of spinal cord and soft tissues.

B. ASSESSMENT OF BACK PAIN

I. Degenerative disease

(a) Plain films

- Plain films are non-specific for the two major degenerative disorders which may be amenable to surgical or other therapy (i.e. degenerative disc disease and spinal stenosis); a large disc protrusion may be present with no plain-film changes; alternatively, the presence of degenerative changes on plain film does not mean that a neurologically significant disc lesion is present.
- Signs of disc degeneration:
  (i)   disc space narrowing;
  (ii) sclerosis of adjacent vertebral end-plates;
  (iii) gas in the disc space;
  (iv) schmorl's nodes (i.e. small, well-defined lytic lesions in the vertebral end-plates);
  (iv) osteophyte formation (i.e. horizontally directed bone spurs on the vertebral end-plates) (*Fig. 20.8*).
- Facet joint changes:
  (i)   osteophyte formation (i.e. bony spurs);
  (ii) enlargement of facets, especially superior articular facets;
  (iii) sclerosis of joint margins;
  (iv) joint space narrowing.
- Other changes:
  (i)   narrowing of intervertebral foramina on oblique film;
  (ii) spondylolisthesis/retrolisthesis seen on lateral film secondary to severe facet joint degeneration.

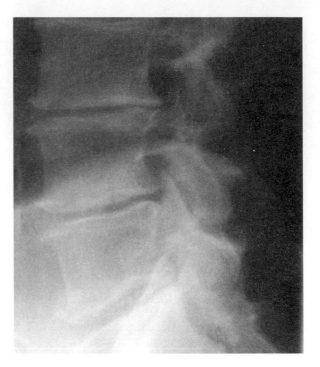

Fig. 20.8   Osteoarthritis of the lumbar spine
Note: • narrowing of the lower 3 disc spaces
         • osteophyte formation at the corners of the vertebral bodies.

(b) MRI (*Fig. 20.9*)

- Investigation of choice for assessment of disc disease and spinal stenosis.
- Disc disease:
  (i) signs of disc degeneration: disc dehydration, disc space narrowing, vertebral end-plate changes;
  (ii) anatomy of disc protrusion: impingement on thecal sac and/or nerve roots, diagnosis and localisation of free disc fragments in the spinal canal or intervertebral foramina.
- Spinal stenosis:
  (i)   narrowing of spinal canal well documented, as well as underlying cause;
  (ii) congenital factors: congenitally narrow spinal canal;
  (iii) degenerative factors: thickening of ligamenta flava, hypertrophy of facet joints, osteophyte formation on vertebral bodies and/or facet joints.

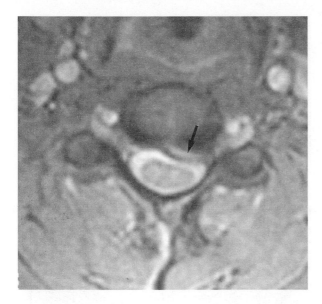

Fig. 20.9   Cervical disc protrusion – MRI
Note: • left postero-lateral disc protrusion (arrow)
        • disc material is compressing the left side of the spinal cord.

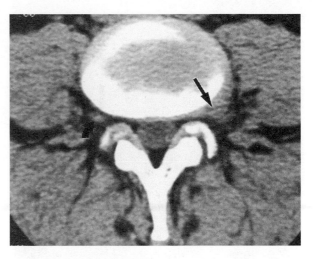

Fig. 20.10   Lumbar disc protrusion – CT
Note: • localised disc protrusion lateral to the left intervertebral foramen impinging on the left nerve root (straight arrow)
        • normal right nerve root (curved arrow).

• Spinal stenosis and disc disease often coexist in the same patient.

(c) CT (*Fig. 20.10*)

• Good for assessment of disc disease and spinal stenosis, though generally less accurate than MRI.

(d) Myelography

• Largely replaced by CT and MRI in the assessment of degenerative disorders.
• Still used in some centres in cases where CT/MRI are equivocal.

2. Spondylosis (i.e. pars interarticularis defect) and spondylolisthesis

Pars interarticularis defects may be congenital or occur as stress fractures in sports such as gymnastics, diving, and fast bowling (cricket). They are most common at L5. Bilateral defects may be associated with spondylolisthesis (i.e. anterior shift of L5 on S1).

(a) Plain films

• Pars interarticularis defects are best seen on oblique views of the lower lumbar spine:
  (i) the complex of overlapping shadows from the superior and inferior articular processes, the pars interarticularis, and the transverse process form an outline resembling that of a Scottish terrier dog.
  (ii) a pars defect is seen as a black line across the neck of the 'dog' (*Fig. 20.11*).
• Spondylolisthesis is graded in severity from grades 1 to 4: each grade represents 1/4 anterior subluxation of L5 on S1 (*Fig. 20.12*).

(b) CT

• Pars interarticularis defects are well shown on CT.
• Scans using a specific angle to 'cut through' the length of the pars interarticularis are extremely sensitive.
• The degree of spinal stenosis and intervertebral foramen narrowing complicating spondylolisthesis are well shown on CT.

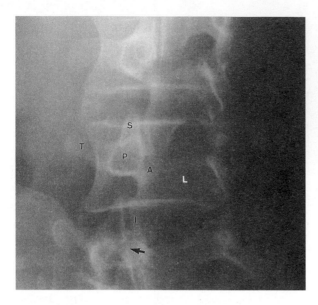

Fig. 20.11   Pars interarticularis defect at L5

Identify the following structures which form the outline of a Scottish terrier dog at L2, L3, and L4:

- transverse process (T)
- superior articular process (S)
- pedicle (P)
- pars interarticularis (A), i.e. the bar of bone seen medial to the pedicle
- inferior articular process (I)
- lamina (L).

There is a pars interarticularis defect at L5 (arrow). This appears to break the 'neck' of the Scottish terrier at this level.

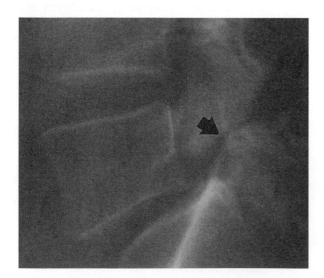

Fig. 20.12   Spondylolisthesis

Note: • bilateral pars interarticularis defects (arrows)
   • forward shift of L5 on S1.

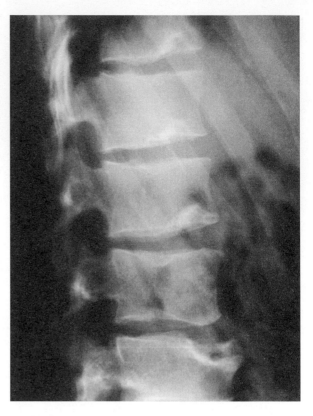

Fig. 20.13   Scheuermann's disease

Note: • irregularity of the anterior two-thirds of the vertebral bodies
   • anterior wedging of the vertebral bodies
   • narrowed irregular disc spaces.

(c) MRI

- Less sensitive than CT or plain films for pars defects.
- Degree of spondylolisthesis and associated spinal stenosis are well shown.

(d) Scintigraphy

- ^{99m}Tc-MDP with SPECT.
- Especially useful to show acute stress lesions of the pars interarticularis in sports injuries.

3. Discitis

(a) Plain films

- Relatively insensitive, i.e. changes are seen after infection has been present for 2 weeks or more.

- Signs:
  (i) disc space narrowing;
  (ii) irregularity of vertebral end-plates.

(b) MRI

- Imaging method of choice.
- Very sensitive for inflammatory changes.
- Complications well shown, e.g. impingement of inflammatory tissue on the spinal canal.

(c) Scintigraphy

- ^{99m}Tc-MDP
- Very sensitive: usually positive from the time of onset of symptoms.

---

4. Scheuermann disease (*Fig. 20.13*)

- Kyphosis ± scoliosis around the thoraco-lumbar junction.

- Involves a minimum of 3 vertebral bodies.
- Anterior wedging of vertebral bodies.
- Irregularity of anterior 2/3 of vertebra end-plates.
- Narrowing and irregularity of intervertebral disc space.
- Multiple Schmorl's nodes.

For notes on general arthropathies which may involve the spine please see Chapter 18.

Further Reading

1. Fagan J, Rogers F. Spinal trauma. *Current Imaging* 1990;**2**:31–41.
2. Kerslake RW, Jaspan T, Worthington BS. Magnetic resonance imaging of spinal trauma. *British Journal of Radiology* 1991;**64**:386–402.
3. Penning L. Obtaining and interpreting plain films in cervical spine injury. In *The Cervical Spine*, 2nd edn. J.B. Lippincot, 1989.
4. Sze G. MR imaging of the spinal cord: current status and future advances *AJR* 1992;**159**:149–159.

21
Paediatrics

A. Neonatal respiratory distress: the neonatal chest
B. Abdominal mass
C. Intussusception
D. Urinary tract infection
E. Pyloric stenosis
F. Non-accidental injury

A. NEONATAL RESPIRATORY DISTRESS: THE NEONATAL CHEST

The normal neonatal chest X-ray has the following features:

* Thymus may be prominent.
* Heart shadow is quite prominent and globular in outline; normal cardio-thoracic ratio up to 65%.
* Air bronchograms may be seen in the medial third of the lung fields.
* Diaphragms normally lie at the level of the 6th rib anteriorly.
* Ossification of the proximal humeral epiphysis occurs at 36 weeks' gestation; visible ossification of this centre implies a term gestation (*Fig. 21.1*).

Most of us approach the chest X-ray of a neonate with some trepidation. It should be borne in mind, however, that the differential diagnosis of neonatal respiratory distress involves only a few abnormalities which tend to give quite typical radiographic patterns, as described below. Remember also that the clinical setting is important, e.g. premature infant: hyaline membrane

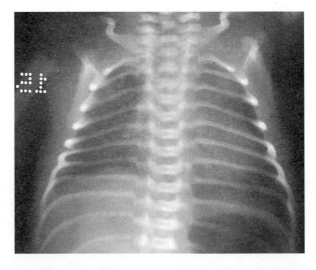

Fig. 21.1   Normal neonatal chest
Note: • prominent superior mediastinal shadow due to the thymus
      • prominent cardiac shadow
      • air bronchograms in the medial thirds of the lung fields.

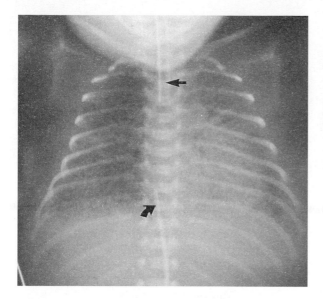

Fig. 21.2   Hyaline membrane disease
Note: • granular pattern through both lungs with air
           bronchograms
        • endotracheal tube (straight arrow)
        • umbilical artery catheter (curved arrow).

disease; Caesarean delivery: retained lung fluid;
term delivery with meconium-stained liquor:
meconium aspiration syndrome. Finally, the first
step in assessing the chest X-ray of a neonate is
to check the position of the various tubes which
may be present:
• Endotracheal tube: tip above carina.
• Umbilical artery catheter: tip in lower
  thoracic aorta away from renal artery
  origins.
• Umbilical vein catheter: tip in lower right
  atrium.
• Intercostal catheter.

1. Hyaline membrane disease (HMD) (*Figs. 21.2 and 21.3*)

• Granular pattern throughout both lungs.
• Air bronchograms.
• Poor pulmonary expansion.
• Complications:
  (i)   pneumothorax;
  (ii) pulmonary interstitial emphysema (PIE):
        air-filled bubbles throughout the lungs;
        high incidence of pneumothorax;
  (iii) patent ductus arteriosus;

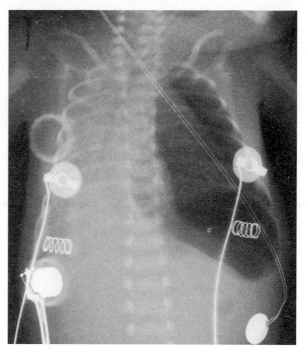

Fig. 21.3   Hyaline membrane disease and pneumothorax
Note: • left tension pneumothorax with enlarged left
           hemithorax and displacement of the heart to
           the right
        • complete opacification of the right lung with air
           bronchograms visible.

(iv) bronchopulmonary dysplasia (BPD)
• Evolves over several days to months
  as a complication of HMD treated
  with positive pressure ventilation.
• Series of changes ranging from severe
  appearances of HMD to persistent
  poor pulmonary expansion and
  marked opacity evolving over several
  weeks to a pattern of over-expansion
  with areas of collapse, fibrosis, and
  bulla formation.

2. Retained foetal lung fluid (also known as transient tachypnoea of the newborn)

• Prominent interstitial pattern with thick-
  ening of lung fissures.
• Small pleural effusions..
• Resolves quickly over 24 hours.

3. Aspiration syndrome

- Over-expanded lungs containing dense, patchy areas of linear atelectasis.
- May be complicated by pneumonia or pneumothorax.

4. Pulmonary oedema

- Cardiomegaly (not a reliable sign in neonates).
- Combination of alveolar and interstitial opacification bilaterally.

5. Neonatal pneumonia

- Range of appearances:
  (i)   lobar consolidation;
  (ii) patchy widespread consolidation;
  (iii) dense, bilateral consolidation may mimic HMD.

6. Pulmonary dysmaturity (Wilson Mikity syndrome)

- Occurs in premature infants.
- Radiological changes and evolution similar to BPD, though with no history of ventilation.

B. ABDOMINAL MASS

The role of imaging for an abdominal mass in a child is as follows:
- Diagnosis and characterisation.
- Treatment planning.
- Guidance of percutaneous biopsy or interventional procedures (e.g. nephrostomy).
- Follow up:
  (i) residual tumour;
  (ii) response to treatment.

1. Ultrasound

- Excellent screening tool: primary investigation of choice.
- Lack of fat in children gives good definition of solid organs and blood vessels.
- Characterisation of masses as cystic, solid, or mixed.

- Ability to image in any desired plane is particularly useful in deciding organ of origin of a mass.
- Can assess blood vessels for vascular invasion as occurs in Wilm's tumour (renal vein and IVC) or hepatoblastoma (portal vein and IVC).

2. Plain films

- Mass may be seen displacing bowel loops.
- Calcification: common in neuroblastoma, though also occurs in other types of tumour.
- Vertebral destruction can occur due to direct invasion by neuroblastoma.
- Chest X-ray:
  (i) pulmonary metastases;
  (ii) paravertebral and mediastinal lymphadenopathy.

3. CT

- CT can be of disappointing quality in children due to a lack of inherent contrast in the form of fat planes between organs.
- Intravenous contrast should be used and sedation is often required.
- CT provides accurate assessment of the contents of a mass, e.g. necrosis, fat, calcification; invasion/displacement of surrounding structures; invasion of the spinal canal as occurs with neuroblastoma.

4. MRI

- MRI has several advantages in children.
- No radiation or iodinated contrast material.
- Excellent soft tissue contrast.
- Multiplanar imaging: the coronal plane is particularly useful in differentiating adrenal from renal masses.

5. Scintigraphy

(a) Renal scintigraphy
- ^{99m}Tc-DTPA.

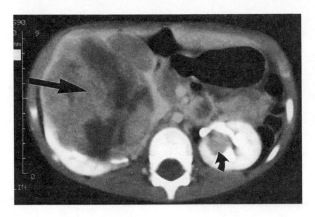

Fig. 21.4 Wilm's tumour – CT
Note: • large mass arising from the right kidney (straight arrow)
• low-attenuation areas within the mass due to necrosis
• small contralateral tumour in left kidney (curved arrow).

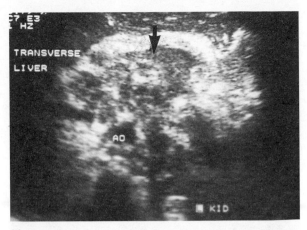

(a)

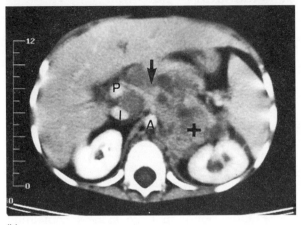

(b)

Fig. 21.5 Neuroblastoma
a) Ultrasound
Ultrasound in the transverse plane shows a large mass (arrow) anterior to the aorta (Ao), with posterolateral displacement of the left kidney.
b) CT
Note: • mass arising from the left adrenal gland (±) continuous across the midline with enlarged pre-aortic lymph nodes (arrow)+
• contrast enhancement in aorta (A), IVC (I), and portal vein (P).

• Useful complement to ultrasound in the assessment of various renal conditions which may present as an adominal mass (e.g. hydronephrosis, pelviureteric junction obstruction, multicystic dysplastic kidney).
• Functional information: differential function, reflux studies, diuretic 'wash-out'.
• Anatomical information: level of obstruction, renal size and outline.

(b) Bone scintigraphy

• ^{99m}Tc-MDP.
• For suspected bony metastases.
• May be accompanied by plain-film review of suspect areas.

A summary is provided below of common abdominal masses in children with their relevant imaging findings.

(i) Multicystic dysplastic kidney:

• Ultrasound: kidney replaced by a collection of non-communicating cysts of varying size.
• Renal scintigraphy: non-function on the affected side.

(ii) Polycystic conditions;

• Autosomal recessive polycystic kidney disease (ARPKD), i.e. infantile and juvenile form.
• Autosomal dominant polycystic kidney disease (ADPKD), i.e. adult form which may occasionaly present in childhood.

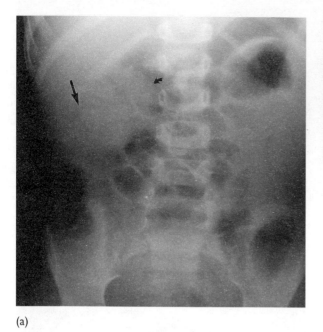

(a)

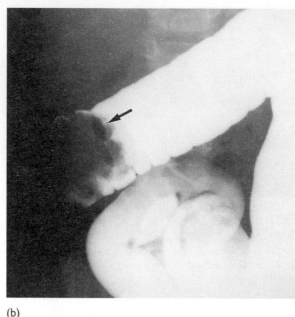

(b)

Fig. 21.6 Intussusception
a) Plain film
Note: • apparent mass in right upper quadrant (straight arrow)
       • intussusceptum shows as a convex opacity outlined by gas; this is the meniscus sign (curved arrow).
b) Contrast enema
The intussusceptum is seen as a filling defect in the transverse colon causing obstruction to the flow of contrast (arrow).

- Ultrasound: in large kidneys containing variable numbers of cysts; cysts may be tiny and innumerable giving the kidney an enlarged hyperechoic appearance.

(iii) Wilm's tumour (nephroblastoma) (Fig. 21.4):

- Ultrasound:
  (i) mass arising from kidney;
  (ii) mass may contain variable cystic areas due to necrosis and occasionally calcification;
  (iii) also look for lymphadenopathy, venous invasion, contralateral tumour, liver metastases.
- CT: mass of variable attenuation arising from the kidney.

(iv) Neuroblastoma (Fig. 21.5):

- AXR: mass in the upper abdomen; significant calcification seen in over 50% of cases.

- Ultrasound:
  (i) mass arising from the adrenal region;
  (ii) heterogeneous echogenicity with areas of necrosis, haemorrhage, and calcification;
  (iii) mass may cross the midline and tends to encase the aorta and IVC.
- CT:
  (i) heterogeneous mass arising from the adrenal region;
  (ii) calcification visible in almost all cases;
  (iii) may cross the midline as above;
  (iv) invasion of the spinal canal.

C. INTUSSUSCEPTION

(a) Diagnosis *(Fig. 21.6)*

I. Plain films

- Small bowel obstruction.

- Meniscus sign due to gas outlining the intussusceptum.
- Relatively gasless right side of abdomen.
- Free air indicates perforation.

2. Ultrasound

- The intussusception is seen as a target-type appearance in cross-section, with a hyperechoic centre due to folds of mucosa and a hypoechoic rim due to swollen, oedematous bowel wall.

3. Contrast enema

- Contrast ceases to flow at the level of the intussusception with the intussusceptum, forming a round, filling defect.
- 'Coiled spring' appearance due to rings of contrast within the folded oedematous mucosa of the intussuscepiens.

(b) Treatment
- Intussusception may be reduced by barium enema; some radiologists perform reduction enema with air or water-soluble contrast.
- Successful reduction is confirmed when contrast enters the terminal ileum.
- Contra-indications to enema reduction:
  (i) shock: the child must be adequately hydrated;
  (ii) perforation: signs of peritonism or free air on AXR.
- Recurrences occur in up to 10% of cases and repeat reduction enema may be performed.
- Surgical consultation prior to reduction enema is mandatory as surgery will be required for:
  (i) failed reduction;
  (ii) perforation;
  (iii) multiple recurrences.

D. URINARY TRACT INFECTION

All children with urinary tract infection should be investigated radiologically so as to:
- Diagnose underlying abnormalities, particularly vesico-ureteric reflux.
- Document renal damage.
- Establish a baseline for subsequent evaluation of renal growth.
- Establish a prognosis.

1. Ultrasound

- Look for urinary tract abnormalities (e.g. pelvi-ureteric junction obstruction, ectopic ureter with hydronephrosis).
- Document scarring of the renal cortex.
- May observe vesico-ureteric reflux, though ultrasound is not reliable for this.

2. Reflux studies

- To document and grade vesico-ureteric reflux and diagnose underlying anomalies such as ectopic ureter or posterior urethral valves:
  (a) Scintigraphic studies.
  (b) Micturating cystourethrogram (MCU).

3. Scintigraphy

(a) ^{99m}Tc-DTPA:
- Quantitates differential renal function.
- Information on renal structure.

(b) ^{99m}Tc-DMSA:
- Most accurate method for documentation of renal scars.

E. PYLORIC STENOSIS

1. Ultrasound

- Has become a very accurate method for diagnosis of pyloric stenosis and usually precludes the need for barium meal.
- The thickened pylorus is seen as a target lesion in cross-section with a thick hypoechoic periphery due to the hypertrophied muscle wall and a hyperechoic centre.
- Pyloric stenosis is diagnosed if the following measurements are obtained:
  (i) total pyloric length >18 mm;
  (ii) total pyloric diameter >15 mm;
  (iii) pyloric muscle thickness >4 mm.

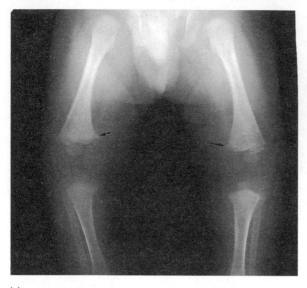

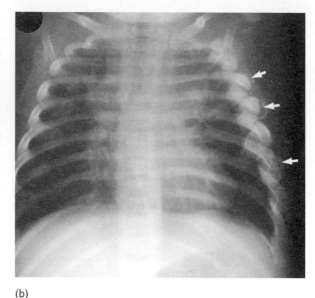

(a)   (b)

Fig. 21.7   Non-accidental injury
a) Lower limbs
There are metaphyseal corner fractures of the lower femora (arrows).
b) Chest
Note callus formation around multiple healing left rib fractures (arrows).

F. NON-ACCIDENTAL INJURY (FIG. 21.7)

Non-accidental injury is a distressing condition for all involved. The importance of making an early diagnosis cannot be overstated and plain films of affected areas, plus skeletal survey (i.e. radiographs of the ribs, skull, and long bones), are important in the diagnostic workup. In considering the diagnosis of non-accidental injury, one should be alert for:

• Fractures inconsistent with the history.
• Multiple fractures at different stages of healing.
• Fractures at unusual sites (e.g. sternum, scapula).

The following patterns may also be seen:

I. Long bones

• Periosteal new bone formation related to prior fractures.
• Metaphyseal or epiphyseal plate fractures.
• Spiral diaphyseal fractures.

2. Ribs

• Up to 80% of rib fractures are occult and may only become visible with healing.
• Posterior rib fractures are particularly suspicious.

3. Skull

• Accidental fractures tend to be linear.
• Non-accidental fractures tend to have the following features:
  (i)   multiple/complex;
  (ii) depressed fractures, especially in the occipital bone;
  (iii) wide fractures (i.e. >5 mm).

4. Other

• A wide range of soft tissue injuries may also occur, including hepatic, splenic, and renal damage, as well as brain damage.

- Subdural haematoma along the falx cerebri in the midline usually indicates severe shaking of the child.

Differential diagnosis of non-accidental injury includes:

- Birth-related trauma.
- Osteogenesis imperfecta.
- Copper deficiency.

Further Reading

1. Bisset GS, III, Kirks DR. Intussusception in infants and children: diagnosis and therapy. *Radiology* 1988;**168**:141–145.

2. Brindle MJ. Children with urinary tract infection; a Critical diagnostic pathway. *Clinical Radiology* 1990;**41**:95–97.

3. Bousvaros A, Kirks DR, Grossman H. Imaging of neuroblastoma: an overview. *Pediatr. Radiol.* 1986;**16**:89–106.

4. Cohen MD, Edwards MK (eds). *Magnetic Resonance Imaging of Children*. B.C. Decker, 1990.

5. Gordon I. Urinary tract infection in paediatrics: the role of diagnostic imaging. *British Journal of Radiology* 1990;**63**:507–511.

6. Newman B (ed.) The pediatric chest. *Radiological Clinics of North America* 1993;**31**:3.

7. Swischuk LE. *Emergency Radiology of the Acutely Ill or Injured Child*, 2nd edn. Williams and Wilkins, 1986.

22
Staging of malignancy

A.   Imaging in malignancy

A. IMAGING IN MALIGNANCY

The roles of imaging in malignancy include:
- Tumour detection.
- Staging.
- Guidance of biopsy.
- Planning surgery and radiotherapy.
- Monitoring of response to therapy.
- Diagnosis of complications of therapy.

This chapter is intended to provide a summary of useful radiological tests in staging of the more common malignancies. Two factors therefore need to be considered: (a) local growth, and (b) pattern of distant spread for each tumour.

(a) *Local growth*

Imaging depends on the pattern of local growth and factors likely to change management, e.g. invasion of organ capsule, invasion of local structures.

(b) *Distant spread*

Imaging depends on the typical pattern of spread, e.g. via lymph channels or blood-borne metastases, and will be aimed at detecting or excluding the more usual types of metastases for each tumour.

First, a few general comments.

(a) Cross-sectional imaging and lymph node size
- Ultrasound, CT, and MRI are generally unable to visualise the internal architecture of lymph nodes.
- As such, size alone remains the only criterion for lymph node involvement with malignancy.
- Lymph nodes of 1.0 cm or greater are considered positive (*Fig. 22.1*).
- Limitations:
  - (i) nodes less than 1.0 cm diameter may have microscopic tumour deposits;
  - (ii) nodes greater than 1.0 cm are not necessarily malignant.

(b) Lung metastases
- As mentioned elsewhere, CT has a higher pickup rate than CXR for pulmonary metastases and as such may be preferable in the initial investigation of tumour with a high rate of spread to the lungs (e.g. testicular carcinoma).
- CXR should also be performed for baseline appearances and for follow-up.

166

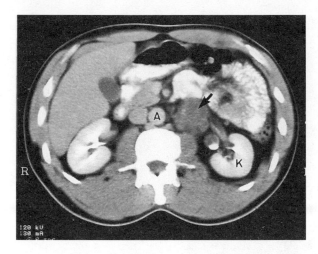

Fig. 22.1 Lymphadenopathy – CT
Note enlarged lymph nodes (arrow) from a primary testicular tumour lying between the aorta (A) and the left kidney (K).

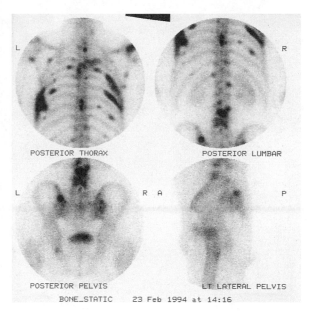

Fig. 22.2 Bone metastases – scintigraphy
Note multiple areas of increased uptake of radiopharmaceutical in the pelvis, spine, and ribs. This indicates multiple sites of increased osteoblastic activity in a pattern typical of disseminated skeletal metastases, in this case from a prostate primary.

(c) Liver metastases
- Ultrasound, CT, MRI, and scintigraphy may all be used for the detection of liver metastases.
- CT scanning performed during dynamic infusion of contrast is probably the most sensitive technique.
- Arterial portography may be used in patients being assessed for possible partial liver resection.

(d) Bone metastases (*Figs. 22.2* and *22.3*)
- Bone scintigraphy (^{99m}Tc-MDP) is generally the most sensitive technique for detection of bone metastases.
- Plain films may be used to assess abnormal or doubtful findings.
- The exception is multiple myeloma in which plain films are more sensitive than scintigraphy.

Having considered the above, the imaging used in the staging of the more common tumours is set out under the subheadings: (a) local growth, and (b) distant spread.

1. Brain

Local growth
- CT.
- MRI.

Distant spread
- Distant metastases from brain tumours are relatively uncommon, so that further imaging is not usually required other than a pre-operative CXR.
- Medulloblastoma/ependymoma may spread to the spine via the CSF: MRI of the spine.

2. Spine

Local growth
- MRI.
- Myelogram with CT.

Distant spread
- Distant metastases from primary spine tumours are uncommon.
- The main exception would be Ewing's sarcoma –
Bone: scintigraphy (^{99m}Tc-MDP)/plain films.
Lung: CXR, CT.

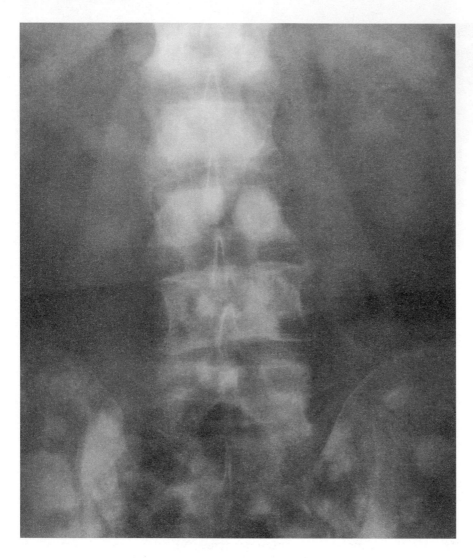

Fig. 22.3 Bone metastases – plain film
There are multiple dense sclerotic lesions throughout the pelvis and spine, in this case due to metastases from a prostate primary.

3. Lung (*Fig. 22.4*)

Local growth
- CXR.
- CT.

Distant spread
- Liver and adrenals: CT.
- Bone: scintigraphy, plain films.
- Brain: CT/MRI.

4. Larynx

Local growth
- Laryngoscopy.
- CT: anatomy of tumour, invasion of laryngeal cartilages, cervical lymph nodes.

Distant spread
- Lung: CXR/CT.

5. Breast

Local growth
- Mammogram.

Distant spread
- Lung: CXR/CT.
- Bone: scintigraphy, plain films.

6. Oesophagus

Local growth
- Barium swallow/endoscopy.

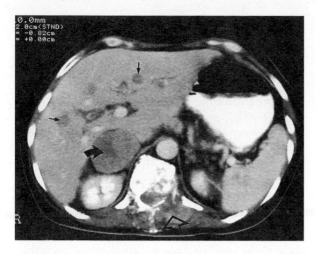

Fig. 22.4 Widespread metastases – CT
Note: • multiple low-attenuation lesions in the liver
(straight arrows)
  • right adrenal mass (curved arrow)
  • paraspinal mass with bone destruction (open
arrow).
This case illustrates hepatic, adrenal, and bone metastases
from a bronchogenic carcinoma.

- CT: invasion of surrounding structures, mediastinal lymph nodes.
- Transoesophageal ultrasound: local invasion and lymph nodes.

Distant spread
- Lung: CXR/CT.
- Bone: scintigraphy, plain films.

7. Stomach

Local growth
- Endoscopy/barium meal.

Distant spread
- Liver: CT.
- Lung: CXR/CT.
- Bone: scintigraphy, plain films.

8. Colon/rectum

Local growth
- Endoscopy/barium enema.

Distant spread
- Liver: CT.
- Lung: CXR/CT.
- Bone: scintigraphy, plain films.

9. Head of pancreas (adenocarcinoma)

Local growth
- CT/ultrasound.
- Cholangiography: ERCP/PTC.

Distant spread
- Liver: CT.
- Lung: CXR.

10. Kidney (renal cell carcinoma)

Local growth
- CT/ultrasound: invasion of adjacent structures, lymphadenopathy, venous invasion.
- Angiogram/cavogram: occasionally used to exclude venous invasion where CT is equivocal.

Distant spread
- Liver: CT.
- Lung: CXR/CT.
- Bone: scintigraphy, plain films.

11. Bladder (transitional cell carcinoma)

Local growth
- Cystoscopy.
- CT: local invasion, pelvic lymph nodes.

Distant spread
- Other sites in urinary tract: IVP.
- Retroperitoneal lymph nodes/liver: CT.
- Bone: scintigraphy, plain films.
- Lung: CXR.

12. Prostate

Local growth
- Transrectal ultrasound and guided biopsy.
- CT: pelvic lymph nodes, invasion of pelvic side wall.

Distant spread
- Bone: scintigraphy, plain films.
- Retroperitoneal lymph nodes: CT.
- Lungs: CXR.

13. Testicle

Local growth
- Ultrasound.

Distant spread
- Retroperitoneal lymph nodes: CT.
- Lung/mediastinal lymph nodes: CT/CXR.

14. Ovary

Local growth
- Ultrasound.

Distant spread
- CT: pelvic and retroperitoneal lymph nodes, ascites, liver metastases.
- Lung: CXR.

15. Cervix

Local growth
- Colposcopy.
- CT/MRI: invasion of local structures, pelvic lymphadenopathy.

Distant spread
- Retroperitoneal lymph nodes, liver: CT.
- Lung: CXR/CT.
- Bone: scintigraphy, plain films.

16. Endometrium

Local growth
- Ultrasound.

Distant spread
- Lungs: CXR/CT.

17. Thyroid

Local growth
- Ultrasound: size of tumour.
- CT: invasion of local strucures, cervical lymphadenopathy, retrosternal spread.

Distant spread
- Lung/mediastinum: CT/CXR.

18. Bone

Local growth
- Plain films.
- Scintigraphy: activity/extent of lesion, exclude multiple lesions.
- CT/MRI: more accurate than plain films for marrow involvement, local invasion, soft tissue involvement.

Distant spread
- Lung: CXR/CT.

19. Multiple myeloma

Skeletal survey, i.e. plain films: more sensitive than scintigraphy in detection of bone lesions in multiple myeloma; typically localised lytic lesions.

20. Lymphoma

(a) *Chest*
- CT.
- CXR.

(b) *Abdomen including liver and spleen*
- CT.
- Ultrasound:
    (i) not as accurate as CT in detection of lymphadenopathy;
    (ii) may be used in follow-up.

(c) *Extranodal disease*
- Gatrointestinal tract: barium studies.
- Bone: scintigraphy, plain films.
- CNS: CT/MRI.

Further Reading

1. Perez CA, Brady LW. *Principles and Practice of Radiation Oncology*, 2nd edn. J.B. Lippincott, 1992.

23
Imaging of AIDS

A. Chest
B. Abdomen
C. Brain

The following is a brief discussion of the use of imaging in the investigation of AIDS.

A. CHEST

The primary investigation of chest problems in the AIDS patient is the chest X-ray. Definitive diagnosis may then be provided by bronchoscopy, biopsy, or bronchoalveolar lavage. Other imaging investigations used include conventional CT with contrast, high-resolution CT (HRCT), and scintigraphy with gallium-67.

I. Infections

(a) Pneumocystis carinii pneumonia (PCP)

- Commonest cause of pneumonia in AIDS.
- Presents with diffuse or perihilar interstitial infiltrates, i.e. a predominantly linear pattern.
- Rapid progression over a couple of days to diffuse bilateral alveolar consolidation which has a 'bat's wing' distribution (*Fig. 23.1*).
- Lymphadenopathy and pleural effusions are uncommon findings.
- Scintigraphy with gallium-67:
    - (i) may provide an early diagnosis where PCP is suspected and the CXR is normal;
    - (ii) PCP produces a diffuse increase in uptake throughout the lungs;
    - (iii) negative in Kaposi's sarcoma.
- HRCT
    - (i) may provide early diagnosis with better delineation of disease activity and distribution;
    - (ii) more specific than CXR, e.g. may distinguish early PCP from other lung lesions.

(b) Mycobacterial infections

(i) Mycobacterium tuberculosis:
- AIDS has been responsible for a marked increase in the incidence of TB in Western society.

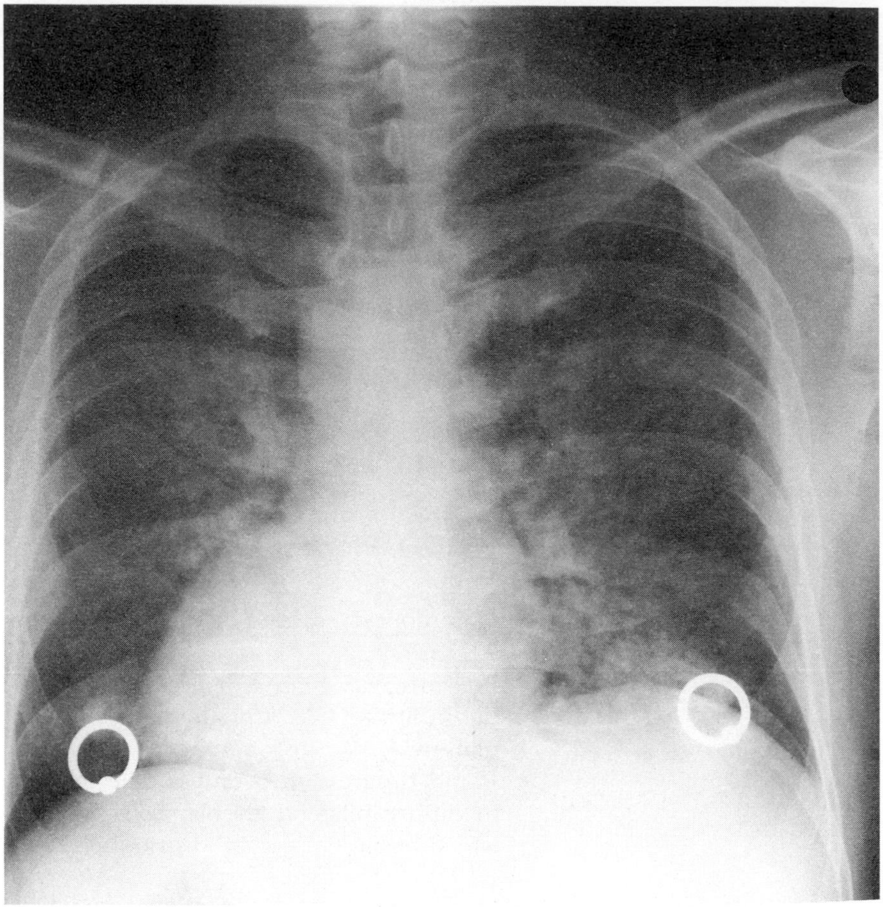

Fig. 23.1 Pneumocystis carinni pneumonia
Note: • typical pattern of widespread, bilateral alveolar opacification
      • nipple rings.

- Two predominant patterns of infection are seen:
    (ii) early HIV infection: resembles non-AIDS TB, i.e. upper lobe infiltration and cavitation;
    (ii) late HIV infection: non-cavitating infiltrates with hilar/mediastinal lymphadenopathy.
- Other investigations – CT with contrast:
    (i) demonstrates lymphadenopathy;
    (ii) pattern of low-attenuation centres in enlarged lymph nodes is seen in TB and other infections, not malignancies.
(ii) Mycobacterium avium-intracellulare (MAI):
- Chest involvement uncommon.
- Hilar/mediastinal lymphadenopathy.

- Non-specific pulmonary infiltrates; occasionally pulmonary nodules.

(c) Fungal infections
- Pulmonary involvement is usually associated with disseminated disease.
- Most common organisms:
    (i)   Cryptococcus neoformans;
    (ii) Histoplasma capsulatum;
    (iii) Coccidioides immitis;
    (iv) Candida albicans.
- Non-specific infiltrates, nodules, cavities, lymphadenopathy.

(d) Bacterial infections
- Most common organisms:
    (i) Staphylococcus pneumonia;

(ii) Haemophilus influenzae.
- Focal consolidation.

2. Neoplasms

(a) Kaposi's sarcoma (KS)

- Pulmonary involvement occurs in 20% of AIDS patients with KS and is usually associated with cutaneous or visceral involvement.
- Bilateral interstitial or alveolar opacification.
- Pulmonary nodules.
- Pleural effusions occur in 30% of cases and may be unilateral or bilateral.
- Lymphadenopathy occurs in 10% of cases.

(b) AIDS-related lymphoma (ARL)

- Predominantly non-Hodgkin's B-cell lymphoma.
- Thoracic involvement uncommon.
- Solitary/multiple pulmonary masses.
- Mediastinal/hilar lymphadenopathy is not a feature of ARL.

3. Other chest lesions

(a) Lymphocytic interstitial pneumonitis (LIP)

- Fine/coarse linear and nodular interstitial infiltrates.
- Areas of focal alveolar consolidation.

(b) Non-specific interstitial pneumonitis (NSIP)

- Diffuse interstitial infiltrates.

4. Differential diagnosis of CXR appearences in AIDS

(a) Diffuse interstitial pattern

- PCP.
- KS.
- LIP.
- NSIP.

(b) Bilateral alveolar pattern

- PCP.

(c) Focal consolidation

- Bacterial infection.
- TB.
- Some fungal infections.

(d) Hilar/mediastinal lymphadenopathy

- TB.
- MAI.
- KS.

(e) Pleural effusion

- KS.
- TB.
- MAI.
- Some fungal infections.

B. ABDOMEN

A wide range of techniques are available for the assessment of abdominal manifestations of AIDS. The type of investigation used will usually be dictated by the presenting symptom (e.g. dysphagia, abdominal pain, jaundice, abdominal mass, gastrointestinal haemorrhage). Methods include:
- Endoscopy with or without biopsy.
- Barium studies.
- ERCP.
- CT/ultrasound.

I. Infections

(a) Candida albicans

- Most common gastrointestinal tract pathogen in AIDS.
- Candida oesophagitis – barium swallow:
  (i) early 'shaggy' appearance to mucosa;
  (ii) later 'cobblestone' appearance, with barium lying between clumps of necrotic debris;
  (iii) ulceration.

(b) Cytomegalovirus (CMV)

- CMV oesophagitis – barium swallow:

(i) ulceration, predominantly in the distal oesophagus;

(ii) ulcers may be large, i.e. over 2.0 cm in diameter.

- CMV gastritis and enteritis: uncommon.
- CMV colitis – barium enema:
  (i) caecum/proximal ascending colon most commonly involved;
  (ii) deep ulceration with swollen irregular mucosa;
  (iii) CT: thickened, oedematous bowel wall.
- CMV cholangitis – ERCP: strictures and dilated segments in common bile duct and intraheptic ducts.

(c) Cryptosporidium

- Most common organism causing AIDS enteritis: small bowel enema:
  (i) increased secretions cause dilution of barium;
  (ii) thickened small bowel wall.
- Cryptosporidium cholangitis – ERCP: same findings as CMV cholangitis.

(d) MAI

- MAI enteritis – small bowel enema:
  (i) small bowel wall thickening;
  (ii) CT: mesenteric lymphadenopathy, small bowel wall thickening.
- Disseminated infection – CT/ultrasound: multifocal abscesses in solid organs, especially the liver.

(e) TB

- TB colitis – barium enema:
  (i) usually involves the caecal area;
  (ii) thickened bowel wall.
- TB oesophagitis – barium swallow:
  (i) deep ulceration;
  (ii) fistula formation.

(f) Herpes simplex

- Herpes oesophagitis – barium swallow: multiple small ulcers.

2. Neoplasms

(a) Kaposi's sarcoma (KS)

- Gastrointestinal tract:
  (i) smooth nodules 0.5–1.0 cm in diameter may occur anywhere from the pharynx to the rectum and may be seen on barium studies of these areas;
  (ii) endoscopic appearances are usually typical.
- Solid organs – CT.
  (i) low-attenuation lesions in liver, spleen, psoas and abdominal wall muscles;
  (ii) extensive lymphadenopathy.

(b) AIDS-related lymphoma (ARL)

- As compared with lymphoma in non-AIDS patients, ARL usually presents with atypical disease patterns such as primary bowel involvement, single large lymph node, higher incidence of focal lesions in liver/spleen.

3. Differential diagnosis of findings of abdominal/gastrointestinal studies in AIDS

(a) Oesophagitis

- Candida albicans.
- Herpes simplex.
- CMV.
- TB.

(b) Gastritis

- CMV.

(c) Enteritis

- Cryptosporidium.
- MAI.

(d) Colitis

- CMV.
- TB.

(e) Nodules in gastrointestinal tract

- KS.
- ARL.

(f)   Lymphadenopathy

- MAI.
- TB.
- ARL.
- KS.

(g)   Liver/spleen lesions

- ARL.
- MAI.
- KS.

(h)   AIDS cholangitis

- CMV.
- Cryptosporidium.

C. BRAIN

CT and MRI are the primary investigations for brain involvement in AIDS. Both investigations may be quite non-specific and multiple types of lesion may co-exist in the one patient. MRI is generally more sensitive than CT.

I.   Infections

(a)   Toxoplasmosis

- Most common CNS infection in AIDS.
- Multiple necrotic abscesses.
- CT/MRI:
  - (i)   multiple lesions throughout the brain associated with oedema;
  - (ii) variable enhancement with contrast.

(b)   Cryptococcus neoformans

- Second most common CNS infection in AIDS.
- Meningitis – CT/MRI often normal; may see communicating hydrocephalus.
- Cryptococcoma: CT/MRI shows solid or ring-enhancing lesion.

(c)   Herpes simplex

- Encephalitis of temporal and inferior frontal lobes.

(d)   J-C papovavirus

- Progressive multifocal leukoencephalopathy (PML).
- Multiple white matter lesions.

(e)   CMV

- Focal areas of infarction/necrosis.

(f)   MAI/TB

- CNS involvement uncommon.
- Cause meningitis or focal inflammatory lesions in the brain.

2.   Neoplasms

(a)   Lymphoma

- Primary CNS lymphoma occurs with much greater frequency in AIDS; it is a rare tumour in the non-AIDS population.
- Non-Hodgkin's lymphoma.
- Second most common cause of focal CNS masses in AIDS after toxoplasmosis.
- CT/MRI:
  - (i)   multiple masses with a predilection for deep white matter of the cerebral hemispheres, corpus callosum, and basal ganglia;
  - (ii) enhancement with contrast, either diffuse or ring enhancement.

(b)   Kaposi's sarcoma

- Rare cause of brain masses.

Further Reading

1.   Federle MP (ed.). Radiology of the immunocompromised patient. *Radiological Clinics of North America* 1992;**30**:3.

Index

abdomen
  abscesses 115
  acute 43–9
  AIDS 173–5
  aortic aneurysm 99–100
  masses 160
  normal 41–2
  trauma 48, 114–15
  X-ray 41–9
abscesses
  abdominal 115
  drainage 72–3
  pulmonary 25–6
absent clavicles 12
absorbed dose, radiation 5
acetabular fractures 140–1
achalasia 109
acoustic
  enhancement 79
  neuroma 93
  shadow 79
acquired immune deficiency
    syndrome (AIDS) 171–5
acute conditions
  abdomen 43–9
  appendicitis 47–8
  cholecystitis 48, 110
  colitis 48
  pancreatitis 110–11
adenocarcinoma 169
ADPKD see autosomal dominant
    polycystic kidney disease
adrenal vein sampling 103
AIDS see acquired immune
    deficiency syndrome
AIDS-related lymphoma (ARL)
    173, 174
air bronchograms 15
ALARA see as low as is reasonably
    achievable
allergic reactions, intravascular
    contrast media 7–9
alveoli 14–16
anaphylactoid reactions 7–9
anechoic 79
aneurysms
  aortic 28, 99–100
  skull 144
angioedema 9
angiography
  techniques 65–9
  abdominal trauma 115
  aortic aneurysm 100
  aortic dissection 100–1
  coronary 95–6
  gastrointestinal bleeding
      112–13
  intracranial lesions 146
  liver mass 117
  magnetic resonance (MRA) 94

peripheral arterial disease 101
  pulmonary 99
  renal 102–3, 119
  stroke 148
  subarachnoid haemorrhage
      144–5
angioplasty 73, 103
ankle joint 134
anterior mediastinal masses 27
antero-posterior (AP) view 41
aorta
  abdominal aneurysm 99–100
  dissection 100–1
  rupture 39
  thoracic aneurysm 28
AP/supine view 11
apophysis 132
appendicitis, acute 47–8
'apple-core' stricture 61
ARL see AIDS-related lymphoma
ARPKD see autosomal recessive
    polycystic kidney disease
artefacts 91, 92
arteriography 65–8
arteriovenous malformation
    (AVM)
  cerebral 75–6, 145
  chest 26
arthritis
  rheumatoid 19, 26, 137
  septic 136
arthrography 68–9, 140
arthropathies, classification criteria
    136–8
as low as is reasonably achievable
    (ALARA) principle 5
asbestosis 19, 32
ascending urethrogram 64
aspiration
  biopsy 71–3
  syndrome 160
asthma 34
atelectasis 38
atherectomy 73–4
atherosclerosis 73
atresia, tricuspid 25
attenuation
  computed tomography 81
  X-rays 1
autosomal dominant polycystic
    kidney disease (ADPKD) 161
autosomal recessive polycystic
    kidney disease (ARPKD) 161
avascular necrosis 135–6, 141
AVM see arteriovenous
    malformation

back pain 154–7
bacterial infections, AIDS 172–3
balloon catheters 73

barium
  enema
    procedure 62
    inflammatory bowel disease
      111–12
    intussusception 163
    Meckel's diverticulum 114
  follow through 61
  meal 59–60
  swallow 59, 109–10
'bat's wing' pattern 15–16
berry aneurysm 94
biceps tendon 140
biliary
  colic 48
  obstruction 62–3
  strictures 76–7
biopsy 71–2, 105
biparietal diameter 126
bladder
  cystoscopy/IVP 120–1
  metastases 169
  trauma 123–4
blow-out fracture 57
BMD *see* bone mineral density
bone mineral density (BMD)
  138–9
bones
  abdominal X-ray 42
  biopsy problems 72
  chest X-ray 13
  growing 131–2
  magnetic resonance imaging 93
  metastases 167, 170
  ossification 131–2
  osteoarthritis 138
  osteoporosis 138–9
  scintigraphy 87, 161
  SPECT scan 87
  spine 149–57
  Sudeck's atrophy 136
  ultrasound 80
bowel
  diverticular disease 113
  inflammatory disease 111–12
  loops 43–6
  obstruction 43–5
  small 45, 59–62, 114
brain
  see also neuro-
  AIDS 175
  magnetic resonance imaging 92,
    93
  metastases 167
  positron emission tomography
    88
breast
  lumps 128–9
  metastases 168
  screening 130

bronchiectasis 36, 105–6
bronchogenic carcinoma
  chest X-ray 35, 36
  computed tomography 105
bronchospasm 9
Buckle (torus) fracture 132

caecal volvulus 45
calcification 42, 55
calculi, salivary glands 58
calf vein thrombosis
  ultrasound 97–8
  venography 68, 98
candida albicans 173
carcinoma
  breast 128
  bronchogenic 35–6, 105
  double-contrast enema 61
  oesophagus 109
  renal cell 118–19
  transitional cell (TCC) 120–2
cardiac
  assessment 26–7
  failure 33
  pacemakers 92
cardiovascular system 8, 95–103
carotid duplex sonography 147–8
catheters, placement 72–3
CCF *see* congestive cardiac
  failure
cell damage 4
central nervous system (CNS)
  142–8
centring, chest X-ray 11
cerebral angiography 67
cerebral function 88
cervical spine 143, 149–52
cervico-thoracic sign 27
cervix 170
chest
  see also pleura; pulmonary
  haemothorax 40
  infections 106
  lung biopsy 72
  pneumothorax 31–2, 40
  respiratory distress 158–60
  respiratory system 104–8
  rib fractures 39, 164
  trauma 38–40
  X-ray (CXR)
    abdominal series 41
    AIDS 171, 173
    hypertension 101–2
    ischaemic heart disease
      95–6
    neonatal 158–9
    plain film 10–40
cholecystitis 48, 110
cholecystotomy 76
claudication 101

clavicles
  absent 12
  cervico-thoracic sign 27
cleidocranial dysplasia 12
clinical practice, imaging in
  95–175
clothing, protective 6
CMV *see* cytomegalovirus
CNS *see* central nervous system
cochlear implants 92
coelic axis 67
'cold' areas 86
colic
  biliary 48
  renal 47
colitis
  acute 48
  ulcerative 112
collapse
  cardiovascular 8
  pulmonary patterns 21–3
  'silhouette sign' 20
colon
  see also bowel
  metastases 169
colour Doppler 80
complicated cyst 118
computed tomography (CT)
  physics of 81–4
  abdomen 114, 115, 160–2
  AIDS 171, 172, 174, 175
  aorta 99–100, 100
  aspiration 72
  biopsy 72
  disc disease 155
  high resolution (HRCT) 105
  liver 116
  pancreas 110–11
  paranasal sinuses 107
  phaeochromocytoma 103
  quantitative 139
  renal system 119, 123
  respiratory system 104–5
  skeletal system 134, 135, 139,
    140
  skull 142–5, 146
  spine
    cervical 152
    disc disease 155
    spondylosis 155
    thoracic/lumbar 153–4
  stroke 147
  subarachnoid haemorrhage 144
congenital heart disease 96–7
congestive cardiac failure (CCF)
  33
consolidation
  pulmonary lesions 14–23
  'silhouette sign' 20
contrast enema 163

contrast media
  computed tomography 81, 83
  intravascular 7–9
  magnetic resonance imaging 93
coronal sutures 51–3
coronary angiography 67–8, 95
coronary artery stenosis 95
craniopharyngioma 55
Crohn's disease 111–12
cryptococcus neoformans 175
cryptosporidium 174
CT see computed tomography
CT arterial portography (CTAP)
  63
CTAP see CT arterial portography
Cushing's disease 103
CXR see chest X-ray
cystic fibrosis 36–7
cystograms 124
cystoscopy/IVP 120–1
cysts
  breast 129
  maternal pelvic 8, 127
cytology, tissue sampling 71
cytomegalovirus (CMV) 173–4

damage, radiation 4–6
decompression drainage 72–3
decubitus film 11
deep vein thrombosis (DVT) 68,
  97–8
degenerative diseases, spine 154–5
delayed union 135
dephasing, magnetic resonance
  imaging 90
depressed fracture 53
deterministic effects, radiation
  damage 4–5
DEXA see dual X-ray
  absorptiometry
diaphragm, rupture 40
diaphysis 131–2
diethyltriaminepentaacetic acid
  (DTPA) 93
digital subtraction angiography
  (DSA) 65–7
disc disease 154–7
discitis 156–7
dislocation, shoulder 140
displacement, fractures 132
diverticular disease 113
Doppler effect 79–80
Doppler ultrasound see ultrasound
dose, radiation 5
double-contrast
  barium enema 61
  barium meal 59–60
drainage procedures 72–3
drop metastases 147

DSA see digital subtraction
  angiography
dual photon absorptiometry 139
dual X-ray absorptiometry
  (DEXA) 139
duodenum 59–60
DVT see deep vein thrombosis
dyspepsia 59
dysphagia 59, 109–10

Ebstein's anomaly 25
echocardiography 7, 80, 96, 107
echogenicity 78
effusions
  ankle joint 134
  elbow joint 133
  knee joint 134
  pleural 30–1
elbow joint effusion 133
embolisation 74–7
embolism, pulmonary 98–9
emphysema 33–4
empyema 32
endometrium, metastases 170
endoscopic retrograde
  cholangiopancreatography
  (ERCP) 62, 116
enemas, bowel 61–2
enteroclysis 60
epiphysis 131–2
ERCP see endoscopic retrograde
  cholangiopancreatography
erect AP 41
erect chest 41
ESWL see extracorporeal shock
  wave lithotripsy
ethmoid sinus 107
expiratory film 11
exposure
  chest X-ray 11
  radiation 4–6
extracorporeal shock wave
  lithotripsy (ESWL) 122
extradural haematoma 142–3

facial trauma 56–7
Fallopian tube catheterisation 77
Fallot's tetralogy 25, 97
fast imaging 94
fat content
  magnetic resonance imaging 91
  ultrasound 79
female reproductive system 126–30
femoral artery 101
femur 140–1
fibrosing alveolitis 106
fibrosis, pulmonary 18–19, 37
fissures, pulmonary 21–2
fixed defects 96
flow, ultrasound 79

flow void 91
foetuses
  lung fluid 159
  morphology 127
  'routine' obstetrical scan 126–7
foreign objects, metal 92
fractures 132–41
  hangman's 152
  hip 140–1
  maxillary 56
  non-accidental injury 164
  seatbelt 153
  skull 51–4, 143
  spine 149–54
  zygomatic 56–7
fungal infections, AIDS 172

^{67}Ga see gallium
gadolinium (Gd) 93
galactography 129–30
gallium (^{67}Ga) scanning 87
gallstone ileus 45
gamma radiation, scintigraphy 85
gantry, computed tomography 81,
  84
Gastrografin 59
gastrointestinal tract (GIT)
  procedures 58–63, 109–17
  AIDS 174–5
  bleeding 112–14
  bowel
    inflammatory disease 111–12
    loops 43–6
    obstruction 46
gated cardiac scan 96
Gd-DTPA 93
genito-urinary (GU) tract
  see also urinary tract;
  procedures 63–5, 77
  bladder
    metastases 169
    trauma 123–4
  urethra 64, 64–5, 123–4
  uterus 126–8
gestational age 126–7
GIT see gastrointestinal tract
gleno-humeral instability 140
glioma 145
gout 138
greenstick fracture 132–3
growing bone 131–2
GU tract see genito-urinary tract
gynaecology 127–8

haematuria, painless 120–2
haemopneumothorax 39, 40
haemothorax 40
hairline fractures 132
hangman's fracture 152
hazards, radiological 4–6

head
    see also intracranial; skull
    trauma 142–4
head of pancreas 169
heart
    see also cardiovascular system
    chest X-ray 12, 26–7, 33
    coronary angiography 95
    echocardiography 7, 80, 96,
        107
    failure 33
    pacemakers 92
helical computed tomography 83–4
hepatic metastases 63, 167
hepatobiliary intervention 76–7
herpes simplex 174, 175
hiatus hernia 28, 109
high attenuation 80
high signal 91
high-frequency scanning 80
high-resolution CT (HRCT)
    105–6
high-risk patients 8–9
hilar disorders 28–30, 104
hip 140–1
histology, tissue sampling 71
HMD *see* hyaline membrane
    disease
Hodgkin's disease 27
hollow organs 41
honeycomb lung 17, 19
hook of hamate, fracture 135
'hot' areas, scintigraphy 86, 87
HRCT *see* high-resolution CT
HSG *see* hysterosalpingogram
hyaline membrane disease (HMD)
    159
hydatid cysts 26
hydrogen atoms 89–90
hyoscine 61
hyperaldosteronism, primary 103
hyperechoic tissues 78–9
hyperosmolar compounds 7
hypertension
    diagnosis of 101–3
    pulmonary 24
hypoechoic tissues 78–9
hysterosalpingogram (HSG) 65

infarcts 96
infections, AIDS 171–5
inflammatory bowel disease
    111–12
inspiration, chest X-ray 11
intercavitary scanning 80
International Commission on
    Radiological Protection
    (ICRP) 4–6
interstitial disease
    chest X-ray 16–19

high-resolution CT 106
oedema 18
pneumonia 37
pneumonitis 173
interventional procedures 71–7, 99
intracerebral haematoma 143
intracranial
    calcification 55
    pressure, raised 56
    space-occupying lesions 145–7
intraduct papilloma, breast 130
intravascular contrast media 7–9,
    93
intravenous pyelogram (IVP) 2–3,
    63–4
    colic 122
    painless haematuria 120–2
    transitional cell carcinoma 119
    trauma 123
intussusception 162–3
iodine 7
ionicity, intravascular contrast
    media 7
IRCP *see* International
    Commission on Radiological
    Protection
ischaemia
    heart disease 95–6
    peripheral 101
IVP *see* intravenous pyelogram

J-C papovavirus 175
jaundice 62, 115–16
jejunal diverticulosis 60
joints
    arthritis
        rheumatoid 19, 26, 137
        septic 136
    arthrography 68–9, 140
    diseases 136–8
    effusions 133–4
    imaging 139–41

Kaposi's sarcoma (KS) 173, 174,
    175
Kerley lines 17, 18
kidney *see* renal
knee
    arthrography 68
    assessment 141
    joint effusion 134
    osteoarthritis 138
KS *see* Kaposi's sarcoma

labral tears 139–40
lambdoid suture 51, 52, 53
large bowel
    barium enema 62
    obstruction 44, 46
Larmor frequency 90

larynx
    metastases 168
    oedema 9
lateral film
    cervical spine 51
    chest 10–11, 13, 14
Le Fort classification 56
lead aprons 6
left atrium 26–7
left lower lobe
    collapse 23
    lesion localisation 21
left upper lobe
    collapse 23
    lesion localisation 21
linear atelectasis 38
linear interstitial pattern 16–17
linear skull fracture 52
LIP *see* lymphocytic interstitial
    pneumonitis
lipohaemarthrosis 135
liver
    mass 116–17
    metastases 63, 167
lobar
    alveolar pattern 15
    collapse 21–3
lordotic view 11
low attenuation 80
low osmolality contrast media 7
low signal 91
lumbar spine 152–4
lungs
    see also pulmonary
    biopsy 72
    chest X-ray 10–40
    CT window 82
    metastases 166, 168
lymph node calcification 42
lymphadenopathy
    AIDS 175
    chest radiography 27
    unilateral hilar enlargement 28
lymphangitis carcinomatosa 18–19
lymphocytic interstitial
    pneumonitis (LIP) 173
lymphoma 170, 175

MAA *see* macroaggregated
    albumen
macroaggregated albumen (MAA)
    98
magnetic resonance angiography
    (MRA) 94, 101
magnetic resonance imaging
    (MRI)
    technique 89–94
    abdomen, paediatric 160
    aorta 100
    brain 175

discitis 157
heart disease 97
intracranial lesions 145–6
kidney 119
physics of 89–94
shoulder 140
skull 6
spine 154–7
spondylosis 156
stroke 148
mal-union 135
malignant disease
see also metastases; neoplasms;
microcalcification 128–30
staging 166–70
mammography 128–30
mandibular fractures 57
margins
abdominal X-ray 42
chest X-ray 21–2
mask film 65–6
maternal pelvic scan 127
maxillary fractures 56
MCU see micturating cysto-
urethrogram
Meckel's diverticulum 114
mediastinum
computed tomography 82, 84
masses 27–9, 104
mesenteric angiography 67
mesothelioma, pleural 32–3
metal foreign objects 92
metaphysis 131–2
metastable energy states 85
metastases
see also malignant disease;
neoplasms;
drop 147
hepatic 63
pleural 33
pulmonary 25, 105
skull 54
staging 166–70
microcalcification, malignant
128–9
microcatheters
genito-urinary intervention 77
neuroradiology 75
micturating cysto-urethrogram
(MCU) 64–5
middle mediastinal masses 27–8
miliary TB 35
monoarthropathy 136–8
MRA see magnetic resonance
angiography
MRI see magnetic resonance
imaging
multicystic dysplastic kidney 161
multiplanar imaging 91
multiple myeloma 54, 170

multiple pulmonary nodules
25–6
musculo-skeletal system
magnetic resonance imaging 93
ultrasound 80
mycobacterial infections, AIDS
171–2
myelography
disc disease 155
technique 69
myocardium
infarcts 95–6
thallium (201T1) exercise test
96

National Health and Medical
Research of Australia,
recommendations 4–6
neck of femur 140–1
necrosis, avascular 135–6
needle biopsy 71–2
neonates
chest X-ray 158–9
pneumonia 160
neoplasms
see also malignant disease;
metastases
AIDS 173, 174, 175
nephroblastoma 162
nephrostomy 77
neurenteric cyst 28
neuroblastoma 161–2
neurogenic tumour 28
neuroradiology 76
nipple discharge 129–30
nodules
interstitial shadowing 17
multiple pulmonary 25–6
solitary pulmonary 25
non-accidental injury, paediatric
164–5
non-aeration, lungs 20
non-specific interstitial
pneumonitis (NSIP) 173
non-union 135
normal X-ray
abdominal 41–2
cervical spine 150
chest 13, 14, 106, 158–9
skull 52
NSIP see non-specific interstitial
pneumonitis
nuclear medicine 6, 85–8

OA see osteoarthritis
oblique view, chest X-ray 11
obstetrical scan, 'routine' 126–7
obstruction
biliary 62–3, 76
bowel 43–5

oedema
allergic 9
interstitial 18
oesophagus
barium swallow 59, 109–10
metastases 168–9
oligaemia, pulmonary 24
OPG see orthopantomogram
orbital fractures 56–7
organogenesis, pregnancy 6
orthopaedics 131–41
orthopantomogram (OPG) 57
osmolality 7
ossification, growing bone 131–2
osteoarthritis (OA) 138
osteoporosis 138–9
ovaries
metastases 170
ultrasound 127–8

PA see posterior-anterior
pacemakers 92
paediatrics 158–65
fractures 132–3
hip pain 141
radiological protection 6
Paget's disease 54, 56
painless haematuria 120–2
pancoast tumour 32–3
pancreas
abdominal X-ray 48, 62
acute pancreatitis 48, 62,
110–11
metastases 169
papilloma, intraduct 130
paralytic ileus 44
paranasal sinuses 107
parotid sialogram 58–9
pars interarticularis defects 87–8,
155–6
patients
high-risk 8–9
radiological protection 6
PCP see pneumocystis carinii
pneumonia
pelvis
obstetric/gynaecological masses
127
trauma 123–4
percutaneous nephrostomy 122
percutaneous transhepatic
cholangiogram (PTC) 62–3,
76, 116
perforation, gastrointestinal tract
45–7
perihilar pneumonia 29
peripheral angiography 67
peripheral arterial disease 101
peristalsis, barium meal 61
pertechnetate 86

PET *see* positron emission
    tomography
phaeochromocytoma 103
phleboliths 42
photon-deficient areas 86
physis 132
piezoelectric effect 78
pituitary adenoma
    magnetic resonance imaging 92
    skull X-ray 55
pituitary fossa 55–6
pivot, tomography 2
placenta, position 126–7
plain abdominal radiography 41–9
plain films
    abdominal trauma 114
    aortic dissection 100
    back pain 154
    bladder/urethra trauma 123
    cervical spine 149–52
    congenital heart disease 96–7
    discitis 156–7
    inflammatory bowel disease 111
    interpretation 10–58
    intussusception 162–3
    paediatric abdominal mass 160
    prostatism 124–5
    renal colic 122
    renal trauma 123
    shoulder 140
    spondylosis 155
    thoracic/lumbar spine 152–3
plane of pivot, tomography 2
plethora, pulmonary 24
pleura
    effusion 30, 107
    thickening 32–3
PMF *see* progressive massive
    fibrosis
PML *see* progressive multifocal
    leukoencephalopathy
pneumocephalus 54
pneumocystis carinii pneumonia
    (PCP) 171
pneumomediastinum 40
pneumonectomy 38
pneumonia
    AIDS 171–3
    chest X-ray 15–16
    interstitial 37
    neonatal 160
pneumonitis 173
pneumoperitoneum 49
pneumothorax
    chest radiography 31–2, 40
    lung biopsy 72
polyarthropathy 136–8
polycystic kidney 161
positron emission tomography
    (PET) 88

post-operative chest X-ray
    non-thoracic surgery 37
    pneumonectomy 38
posterior mediastinal masses 28
postero-anterior (PA), chest X-ray
    10
precession 90
pregnancy, radiological protection
    6
primary hyperaldosteronism 103
probes, ultrasound 80
progressive massive fibrosis (PMF)
    19
progressive multifocal
    leukoencephalopathy (PML)
    175
projections
    chest X-ray 10–11
    skull X-ray 51
prostate, metastases 175
prostatism 124–5
protection, radiological 4–6
psychiatric assessment, positron
    emission tomography 88
PTC *see* percutaneous transhepatic
    cholangiogram
pulmonary
    angiography 67, 99
    arterial hypertension 24
    collapse patterns 21–3
    dysmaturity 160
    embolism 98, 98–9
    lesion localisation 20–1
    metastases 25, 105, 166
    nodules 25–6
    oedema 9, 160
    oligaemia 24, 97
    plethora 24, 97
    vascular patterns 23–4
    venous hypertension 24
pyelogram
    intravenous (IVP) 63
    retrograde 64
pyloric stenosis, paediatric 163–4

quantitative computed tomography
    139
quantitative ultrasound 139

radiation
    dose units 5
    hazards 4
    protection 5–6
radio-pharmaceuticals 85
radio-ulnar joint 69
radiofrequency (RF) pulse 90
radiography
    see also computed tomography
        (CT); normal X-ray; X-rays
    conventional 1–2

densities 1–2
    sectional 2–3
radiological hazards 4
radionuclides 85–6
raised intracranial pressure 56
reactions, contrast media 7–9
receiver coils 90
rectum 169
recurrent dislocation, shoulder 140
reflux studies, paediatric 163
renal
    angiography 67, 102
    artery stenosis 102
    calculus 120, 121, 122
    colic 47, 122
    mass 118–20
    trauma 123
renal cell carcinoma
    bowel obstruction 44
    imaging techniques 169
    ultrasound 118–19
renal vein renins 103
renins, renal vein 103
reproductive system, female
    126–30
respiratory system
    imaging techniques 104–8
    neonatal distress 158–60
resuscitation 8–9
retained foetal lung fluid 159
retrograde pyelogram 64
retroperitoneal mass 44
retrosternal goitre 27
'reversed bat's wing' pattern 16
RF pulse *see* radiofrequency pulse
rheumatoid disease 19, 137
    nodules 26
ribs
    fractures 39
    non-accidental injury 164
right atrium, enlargement 26
right lower lobe, collapse 21
right middle lobe, collapse 21–2
right upper lobe, collapse 21
risk factors, intravascular contrast
    media 8
rotator cuff disease 140
'routine' obstetrical scan 126–7
rupture
    thoracic 40
    urethral 125

sagittal suture 53
salivary glands 58–9
Salter Harris fracture classification
    132–3
samples
    adrenal vein 103
    size, biopsy 71
sarcoidosis 17, 19, 29, 35–6

Scheuermann's disease 156–7
scintigraphy 85–8
  abdominal abscess 115
  cholecystitis 110
  discitis 157
  gastrointestinal bleeding 113–14
  hypertension 102
  liver
    jaundice 116
    mass 117
  Meckel's diverticulum 114
  paediatric
    abdominal mass 160–1
    urinary tract infection 163
  pars interarticularis defects 156
  phaeochromocytoma 103
  respiratory system 106–7
  stress fractures 134
  thallium (201Tl) exercise test
    96
seatbelt fracture 153
sectional radiography 2–3
segmental alveolar pattern 15
Seldinger technique 73
sentinel loops 44
septic arthritis 136
shadowing
  alveolar 14–16
  interstitial 16–19
shoulder
  arthography 68
  assessment 139–40
  high frequency ultrasound 80
sialography 58–9
sigmoid volvulus 44–5, 46
'silhouette sign' 20
silicosis 19
simple renal cyst 118
single photon emission computed
  tomography (SPECT) 87–8
single-contrast 60
sinus disease 107
skeletal system 131–41
  see also bones; skull; spine;
  non-accidental injury 164–5
skull
  non-accidental injury 164
  trauma 51–4
  vault thickening 56
  X-ray 51–8
SLAP see superior labrum anterior
  to posterior
slip-rings 83
small bowel
  enema 61–2, 114
  obstruction 45
solid organs
  normal abdominal X-ray 42
  ultrasound 80
solitary pulmonary nodule 25

space-occupying lesions,
  intracranial 145–7
SPECT see single photon emission
  computed tomography
spine
  cervical 143, 149–52
  computed tomography 152–4
  lumbar/thoracic 152–4
  magnetic resonance imaging 92,
    93
  metastases 167
  myelography 69
  spondylosis 87–8, 155–6
  trauma 149–54
spiral computed tomography 83–4
spondylolisthesis 155–6
spondylosis 87–8, 155–6
spread, malignancy 166–70
staging of malignant disease
  166–70
standard X-ray series
  abdominal 41
  skull 51
stenosis
  coronary artery 95
  renal artery 102
  therapies 73–4
stents, vascular 73
stochastic effects 4
stomach
  see also gastrointestinal (GI) tract
  barium meal 59–60
  metastases 169
strangulated hernia 45
stress fractures 134–5
stroke 147–8
subarachnoid haemorrhage 144–5
subdural haematoma 143
subtle fractures 132–5
Sudeck's atrophy 136
superior labrum anterior to
  posterior (SLAP) 139
sutures 51–34

201Tl see thallium (201Tl)
  exercise test
T1/T2 relaxation 90–1
TB see tuberculosis
99mTc see technetium
TCC see transitional cell
  carcinoma
'teardrop' fracture 151–2
technetium (99mTc) 85–6
temporo-mandibular joint 57
temporo-parietal suture 52
tendonitis 140
tension pneumothorax 31
testicle 169–70
thallium (201Tl) exercise test 96

thoracic spine 152–4
thrombolysis 73–4
thymus 27
thyroid 170
TIA see transient ischaemic attack
TIPS see transjugular intrahepatic
  portosystemic shunt
tissue densities
  computed tomography 81
  text:tissue sampling 71–2
tomography
  computed (CT) see computed
    tomography (CT)
  conventional 2–3
  positron emission (PET) 88
  single photon emission
    computed (SPECT) 87, 88
torus fracture 132
Towne's view 51–3
toxoplasmosis 175
transabdominal ultrasound 127
transient ischaemic attack (TIA)
  147–8
transient tachypnoea of the
  newborn 159
transitional cell carcinoma (TCC)
  169
  intravenous pyelogram 119
  painless haematuria 120–1
transjugular intrahepatic
  portosystemic shunt (TIPS)
  76
transrectal probes 80
transvaginal ultrasound 128
trauma
  abdominal 48, 114–15
  bladder/urethra 123–4
  chest
    computed tomography 105
    radiography 38–40
  facial 56–7
  head 142–4
  monoarthropathy 136
  non-accidental injury 164–5
  pelvic 123–4
  pleural thickening 32
  pneumocephalus 54
  renal 123
  skull 51–4, 142–4
  spine 149–54
triangular fibro-cartilage complex
  69
tricuspid atresia 25
99mTc-DTPA, ventilation/perfusion
  lung scan 98
99mTc-MAA, ventilation/perfusion
  lung scan 98
tuberculosis (TB)
  AIDS 174
  CXR appearance 19, 34–5

tumour spread, staging 166–70
tungsten target 1

ulcerative colitis 112
ultrasound 78–80
  abdomen 115
  aortic aneurysm 99
  breast lumps 129
  carotid duplex sonography
      147–8
  cholecystitis 110
  deep venous thrombosis 97–8
  gynaecology 127–8
  hypertension 102
  intracranial lesions 146–7
  intussusception 163
  liver
    jaundice 115
    mass 116–17
  obstetrical 126–7
  paediatric
    abdominal mass 160–2
    pyloric stenosis 163–4
    urinary tract infection 163
  painless haematuria 122
  pancreatitis 110–11
  peripheral arterial disease 101
  prostatism 124–5

quantitative 139
renal mass 118–19
renal trauma 123
respiratory system 107
shoulder 140
venography 68
urethrograms
  ascending 64
  bladder/urethra trauma 123–4
  micturating cysto- 64–5
urinary tract 118–25
  paediatric 163
uterus, ultrasound 126–8

varicocele embolisation 77
vascular
  embolisation 74, 76
  markings, skull 52–3
  patterns, pulmonary 23–5
  stents 73
  therapies 73–6
venography
  deep venous thrombosis 98
  technique 68
ventilation/perfusion lung scan
    98–9
vertebra see spine
viewing, radiographs 11–13

von Hippel-Landau syndrome 147

Wegener's granulomatosis 26
Wilm's tumour 162
Wilson Mikity syndrome 160
window settings 81–2
wrist
  arthrogram 69
  assessment 139

X-rays
  abdominal 41–9
  chest 10–40, 95–6, 171
  computed tomography 81–4
  conventional radiography 1–2
  normal
    abdominal 41–2
    cervical spine 150
    chest 13, 14, 106, 158–9
    skull 52
  sinus 107
  skeletal system 131–7
  skull 51–8
  spine 149–57

Z-plane, computed tomography 84
Zenker's diverticulum 109–10
zygomatic fractures 56–7